"DOWAGER'S HUMP," SHRINKING WITH AGE, BONES THAT BREAK EVEN BEFORE YOU FALL . . .

OSTEOPOROSIS

The symptoms of osteoporosis afflict millions of people. Many think it's a woman's disease, but men are not immune. Who is at greatest risk? Why? The answers are vitally important for the prevention and treatment of this devastating disease. Now, here are the facts you need to save your health.

Doctors have known about osteoporosis for over a century, yet only recently has the disease begun to receive public attention. In *Osteoporosis*, Margot Joan Fromer shows how to delay the onset of the disease. With care, attention to diet, a moderate exercise program, and a reasonable amount of extra calcium, many people can stand up straighter and longer—into their old age.

OSTEOPOROSIS

MARGOT JOAN FROMER, R.N.

PUBLISHED BY POCKET BOOKS NEW YORK

Another *Original* publication of POCKET BOOKS

POCKET BOOKS, a division of Simon & Schuster, Inc.
1230 Avenue of the Americas, New York, N.Y. 10020

ISBN: 0-671-54687-2

First Pocket Books printing January, 1986

10 9 8 7 6 5 4 3 2 1

POCKET and colophon are registered trademarks
of Simon & Schuster, Inc.

Printed in the U.S.A.

Contents

List of Illustrations

PREFACE

Although doctors have known about osteoporosis for over a century, many people think it's a new disease because it has so recently begun to receive public attention. Only within the past few years have we become aware of how devastating osteoporosis is and how easy it is to retard its progress. Osteoporosis is still incurable, but it can be controlled to a significant extent.

Medicine has discovered the link between this great crippler of old people, menopause, and calcium intake. This book describes what osteoporosis is, what causes it, and what you can do to stave it off for as long as possible.

Although almost *everyone* gets osteoporosis sooner or later, it is possible now to delay the onset of the disease by taking a few simple measures, most of which do not require a physician's direction. With a bit of care and attention to diet, a moderate exercise program, and a reasonable amount of extra calcium, people can stand up straighter and longer into their old age, and they can, to a great extent, avoid that most frightening consequence of osteoporosis: the broken hip which often results in a life of crippled immobility in a wheelchair.

I am most grateful to the women who invited me into their homes, told me about their experiences with osteoporosis, and shared their feelings with me. Without their forthrightness, this book would not be what it is.

MARGOT JOAN FROMER
SILVER SPRING, MARYLAND

Chapter One

OSTEOPOROSIS: WHAT IT IS

*I*t's called "dowager's hump" and the "little old lady" syndrome. It's more prevalent in women than men, but it happens sooner or later to almost everyone who grows old— sooner to women than to men. It can cause a hip or wrist fracture from a simple fall, and it decreases life expectancy because hip fracture is the leading cause of accidental death in people aged 75 and over and the second leading cause of accidental death in people aged 45 to 74.

It is osteoporosis, and its definition is a decrease in the amount of bone in your body.

Your bony skeleton is about ten percent of body weight, although the total skeletal mass decreases with age, and this decrease diminishes bone strength. However, the total amount of bone a person has is not necessarily the main determinant of osteoporosis and consequent fracture risk because that would mean that the smaller the person, the more likely he or she is to break a bone, and there is no evidence that this is true. The main determinant of bone strength and fracture risk is the amount of bone in the bone; that is, the density of bone tissue.

The number and shape of a person's bones does not change over the years; rather, over time each bone contains less bone tissue, which becomes softer and spongier. Thus, the skeletal structure, on which muscles, tendons, and all the other tissues and organs of the body depend for support, weakens.

The chemical composition of the bones remains unchanged, so osteoporosis is not like a car rusting away with age.* Instead, bone tissue is destroyed faster than it can be replaced by the formation of new whole bone. It's rather like a frame house that looks fine from the outside but is being eaten away by termites from within. Even that analogy is not altogether precise because some people with advanced osteoporosis *don't* look fine from the outside. They grow shorter and frailer, almost as if they were caving in on themselves. They literally waste away with age.

There are two major kinds of bone: cortical and trabecular. The cortical bone is a dense compacted mass of bone tissue that forms the external or covering layer of bones. Trabecular bone (figure 1) resembles a honeycomb, it consists of lattices of spongy bone tissue filled with embryonic bone and bone marrow. It makes up about 20 percent of the total skeletal mass. Cortical bone (figure 2) derives its strength from the compactness of the tissue itself, and trabecular bone is strong because of its intricate architecture.

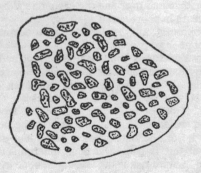

FIGURE #1
Cross Section of Trabecular Bone

---

*That description fits a condition known as osteomalacia in which the *amount* of bone remains normal, but the mineral content decreases, and there is a delayed mineralization of new bone.

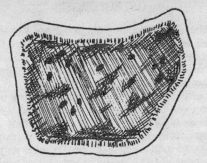

FIGURE #2

Cross Section of Cortical Bone

All bones contain both types of tissue, but the proportion changes from bone to bone. The long bones (those in the arms, legs, fingers, and toes) are more cortical than trabecular, and the flat bones (the vertebrae, facial bones, pelvic bones, and the like) are more spongy than dense.

Osteoporosis affects both types of bone, but the results are different. Long bones appear healthy until they suddenly snap, usually at the neck of the bone where it narrows to form the head. A hip fracture, one of the most common results of osteoporosis, is not really a fracture of the pelvis but is rather a snapping off of the head of the femur, the long bone that runs from the knee to the pelvis. The other common accident of osteoporotic long bones is the Colles fracture, in which the neck of one of the two bones that run from the elbow to the hand, the radius and/or the ulna, breaks. The break usually occurs at the wrist end.

When osteoporosis attacks trabecular bone, it causes spinal curvature (dowager's hump), loss of height, and fractures of the vertebrae, some of which may be hardly noticeable on an X-ray but are still excruciatingly painful.

Bone is composed of protein and a variety of minerals, the two most important of which are calcium and phosphorus, bound together in an interlocking grid. Like most other tissues of the body, bone undergoes a constant process of buildup and breakdown because cells die and new cells are manufactured to replace the dead ones. All cells in all tissues have a finite life expectancy, the longevity varying with the type of cell. Most cells replace themselves,* but the replacement process slows with age. This is one of the causative factors in osteoporosis. It is also why the healing of *all* tissue takes longer in old people than in young ones.

The process by which new bone replaces the old is called remodeling: old bone continuously breaks down (resorbs), and new bone is formed to replace it or add to it. In children and adolescents more bone is formed than is resorbed; your bone mass (the total amount of bone) reaches its peak somewhere between 30 and 40 years of age. During adult life, bone remodeling becomes a delicate balancing act which is affected by age, sex, weight, race, body build, diet, physical activity, and other variables. For example, when you gain weight, the bone responds to the increased load by stimulating growth of new bone tissue because it senses the stress of the added weight.

New bone is also formed in reaction to the resorption of old bone. Bone breakdown cells, called osteoclasts, dig microscopic grooves and craters on the bone surface as they destroy bone tissue. If resorbing bones were magnified, they would look like potholed pavement after a hard winter.

Osteoblasts, or bone *forming* cells, respond to the unevenness in the surface of the bone by building new bone tissue to smooth out the surface. Then, other pits and craters appear, and the osteoblasts go to work again.

Bone mineralization, the process by which the bone forming cells produce the protein and stimulate the placement of mineral crystals, takes about three or four months. New bone lasts anywhere from three to ten years; it is then slowly resorbed.

Bone remodeling continues throughout your life, but as you grow older, more bone is resorbed than is produced, causing a slow but steady diminution of bone mass. This is called osteoporosis.

Osteopenia is a decreased volume of mineralized bone tissue, and osteoporosis is a reduction in bone volume as a

---

*Among the notable exceptions are brain cells and some, but not all, nerve cells.

result of an irreversible decrease in mineralized bone. In other words, osteopenia is the process, and osteoporosis is the result.

Measuring total bone volume is more difficult than one might think. An X-ray of bone simply shows the character of the tissue to some extent; it cannot show how much tissue there is in relation to the number of bones. The X-ray can show the density of bone (though again, only to a limited extent), but total bone mass cannot be measured by radiograph alone.

According to Z. F. G. Jaworski in "Physiology and Pathology of Bone Remodeling": "Unfortunately, in order to assess the total bone volume we have to rely, often for the sake of convenience, on methods that estimate it or its changes indirectly, by measuring the bone mineral content or the volume of mineralized bone. Such methods cannot discriminate between the total and mineralized bone volumes or between changes in total bone volume and remodeling space."

In other words, diagnosing early osteoporosis, as well as the progress of the later stages of the disease, is almost purely guesswork. Jaworski does, however, suggest two indirect ways to measure reduced bone volume. The first is the statistical norm for age and sex. That is, an individual is compared to an average population. The second method is the volume-dependent fracture threshold. This is an almost absolute standard in the same way that a certain amount of steel and concrete is necessary to maintain the structural integrity of a bridge. It means that a certain amount of bone tissue is absolutely necessary to maintain a particular bone's structural integrity, and when there is less bone than this necessary volume, the threshold has been crossed and the bone will break.

However, total bone volume may not be the only contributing factor to osteoporosis, and the matter becomes complicated. We shall discuss this in more detail later.

All bones are composed of three different layers, called envelopes, all of which have the same cellular composition (that is, bone breakdown and bone forming cells), but different anatomical construction. Their growth rate also differs. The growth rate of bones, particularly long bones, is much like the annual growth pattern of trees, which can be measured by examining the growth rings after the tree is felled. In good years, when there is lots of rainfall and sunlight, the tree grows faster and the growth ring is wider. In lean years, when there is a drought or forest fire, the growth ring is narrow, indicating slow growth.

So too with bones. The inner ring (the endosteal envelope) is the closest to the marrow cavity and is the first to break down in early adulthood. This is the beginning of the diminution of bone mass that continues, at varying rates, until death.

The middle ring (the intracortical envelope) remains in fairly good balance throughout life, with one notable exception: prolonged inactivity, such as being confined to bed or an extremely sedentary lifestyle, causes the intracortical envelope to break down. Since this is the thickest part of the bone and contributes the most to the skeletal support system, prolonged inactivity is a serious matter.

The outer layer (the periosteal envelope) is where the most rapid growth takes place during childhood and adolescence. This process reverses as the person grows older. Osteoporosis has a profound effect on the anatomical structure of this outer envelope because it is the densest and most compact of the three layers.

Bone loss will probably, although not necessarily, lead to bone fracture, but all bone fractures are not a consequence of bone loss. However, especially in older people, bone fractures from causes other than osteoporosis may hasten or even initiate the osteoporotic process because of the necessary prolonged immobility of the bone while the fracture heals.

In terms of large numbers of people, or even total population groups, there is a high correlation between bone loss and bone fracture. In individual cases, however, this may not be true. Jaworski thinks there may be several reasons for this apparent contradiction: first, older people may fall because they have impaired nerve-muscle coordination, not because their bones are weak. Second, there may be spaces of poorly mineralized bone within a bone that is generally adequately mineralized. This makes those patches of mineral-poor bone particularly vulnerable to fracture. Third, the bone may break because of some other disease process such as osteomalacia, osteosarcoma (cancer), Paget's disease (chronic inflammation and thickening of the bone), or osteomyelitis (a bone infection). Therefore, says Jaworski, "It may be preferable to reserve the term 'osteoporosis' for the reduction of total bone volume to distinguish it from the bone fragility syndrome of aging."[1]

Bones evolve from embryonic cartilage that converts to bone during pre-natal life and the early years after birth. Bone growth is regulated by specific hormones and other substances as well as by weight and physical activity. Some of the substances that affect bone are:

• Parathyroid hormone (PTH) which regulates the production of calcium and Vitamin D. It also controls the amount of calcium absorbed by the intestines. PTH stimulates bone resorption which in turn releases stored calcium into the bloodstream. Thus, an overabundance of PTH is harmful because it causes bone to break down.

• Vitamin D, which is really a hormone rather than a vitamin. Vitamin D is stored, in a semi-active state, in the liver. From there it is transported to the kidneys in an active form. It increases the absorption of calcium by the intestines, and it resorbs calcium through the kidneys. In short, Vitamin D regulates both circulating and stored calcium levels and can even remove it from bones if they become too calcium-rich. Because calcium is such an important component of bone, it is *crucial* to maintain adequate levels of Vitamin D.*

• Calcitonin, a hormone released by the thyroid gland. It is believed to inhibit the activity of bone breakdown cells, osteoclasts, thereby slowing bone resorption. It also protects bone from the dissolving effects of PTH and activated Vitamin D.

• Estrogen, produced by the ovaries before menopause and by other body tissues, most especially fat tissue, after

---

*See the chapter on diet for a list of foods that are high in calcium and Vitamin D.

menopause. Estrogen is the substance most closely associated with osteoporosis, and diminished levels of this female hormone is believed to be one of its primary causes. Estrogen has an inhibitory effect on adrenal hormones (those produced by the adrenal glands, such as androgen, a male sex hormone). Thus, when estrogen production is reduced and changed at menopause,* there is less to curb the production of adrenal hormones which are believed to be associated with osteoporosis, although the mechanism is not fully understood. Researchers think that adrenal hormones have a direct effect on osteoclasts, thus speeding up bone resorption.

• Progestogen (commonly called progesterone), also produced by the ovaries before menopause, protects bone by inhibiting the negative action of adrenal hormones to some extent. Since progestogen production ceases even earlier than ovarian estrogen production, there is a greatly diminished counterbalancing effect after menopause, and the osteoporotic process can increase.

• Growth hormone, which stimulates bone growth. It is unclear what role this hormone plays in the remodeling of adult bones, but it seems reasonable to assume that osteoporotic postmenopausal women are less able to produce growth hormone than non-osteoporotic postmenopausal women.

Women have a much higher incidence of osteoporosis than do men, especially after menopause. The reason for this remains a source of speculation, but it is generally believed that the diminution of ovarian function has a profound effect on several glands—and the hormones they produce—which in turn affects bone remodeling.

Significant bone loss generally starts at menopause in women** and somewhat later in men. It continues to the end of life at the rate of approximately one percent per year in women and one half of one percent in men. Fifty percent of

---

*See the chapter on estrogen replacement therapy for a more complete discussion of estrogen and its association with osteoporosis.
**The average age for menopause is 50, and the age range is 45 to 55 years.

all women have osteoporosis by age 70, and one hundred percent of them have it by age 90. About fifty percent of all men have osteoporosis by age 80. The cause of the disease in men is unknown, but it may be due to a decrease in testicular or adrenal androgen production.

The rate at which bone is lost also differs in men and women. Women experience an extremely rapid loss in the first decade after menopause, and then the rate of loss slows somewhat. In fact, women lose dense bone about twice as fast as men. The difference in the rate of spongy bone loss is even greater, which is why old women appear to shrink faster and to a greater extent than old men. Men start out with denser bones than women, so it's only natural that they should experience less severe bone loss, but after age 70 or so, men and women lose bone at more nearly the same rate, although women *appear* to shrink faster because they had a decade or so "head start" on men.

Bone mass can be determined at certain sites by X-ray, a procedure called densiometry,* and bone biopsy, in which a small sample of bone is surgically removed and the cells examined under a microscope. In women, bone status is measured in years since menopause, whereas in men it is measured by chronological age. This difference in measurement method is not unfair, and it is not sexist; it is simply the most practical procedure in light of the fact that osteoporosis has a more definite onset in women, whereas in men there is no precise onset.

At menopause, women's calcium requirements increase from 500 to 600 mg. a day to 1200 to 1500 mg. a day. There is no precise age at which men should start increasing their calcium intake, although they should certainly be doing so by age 70.

The presence or absence of estrogen seems to be a major factor in the osteoporotic differences between men and women. Men *do* have estrogen; it is converted from adrenal androstenedione (a form of androgen), and the levels of estrogen circulating in the bloodstreams of men under age 60 is higher than circulating estrogen in postmenopausal women—

---

*This will be described in the chapter on diagnosis and treatment.

unless they are taking replacement estrogens. There is no clear explanation as to why men get osteoporosis at all and why the onset should be so different from that in women.

Osteoporosis affects different population groups in different ways. In the United States one of the most severely affected groups is white menopausal women who are small-boned, thin, and who smoke. They are at extremely high risk for osteoporosis (some sources say they are at the highest risk), whereas American blacks, especially men, are at lowest risk. Black people have a larger skeletal volume than do white people, and their bones contain more bone tissue. Black women lose less bone than do white women, and they lose it at a slower rate. Consequently, they have fewer fractures. No one knows why there is this pronounced difference between blacks and whites.

Orientals in the United States (those of Chinese and Japanese ancestry) have smaller skeletons than Caucasians, and they lose bone at a faster rate. One speculation about the reason for this is that Orientals may have a lactose intolerance and therefore have a lower lifetime calcium intake. There is, however, no clinical proof of this.

Some osteoporosis is normal in everyone who ages. It is considered pathological (meaning disease is present and it's sometimes referred to as accelerated osteoporosis) when the degree of bone loss is greater than normal. The problem in defining "normal" and "accelerated" is knowing what degree of bone loss is normal at any particular age. It is fairly easy to measure statistical averages on large population groups, but "average" does not necessarily mean "normal" because it is not unknown for large groups of people to suffer from a disease, making the disease state *average* but certainly not *normal*. There are no precise lines of demarcation, and every orthopedic specialist has a different set of criteria to determine when osteoporosis moves into the acceleration lane. It is virtually impossible to establish normal levels because there are so many variables in age-related bone loss; for example: thyrotoxicosis (a disease of the thyroid gland); treatment with thyroid extract for hypothyroidism; various forms of malabsorption of nutrients, particularly minerals; prolonged ingestion of aluminum-containing antacids (such as Maalox and Gelusil); kidney failure; and collagen diseases* such as lupus erythematosus, rheumatoid arthritis, and the like.

There is also no absolute proof that people lose bone mass as they age, although it seems safe to say that the vast majority do—sooner or later.

In addition to diminution of ovarian function at menopause, there are other chemical changes that signal the onset of osteoporosis: high levels of calcium and hydroxyproline (a complex protein) in the urine indicate a negative bone balance, that is, that more bone is being resorbed than produced. The presence of alkaline phosphatase (a mineral) in abnormally high levels in the bloodstream indicates osteomalacia or some other bone pathology, possibly osteoporosis. The principal metabolic cause of osteoporosis is malabsorption of calcium, although the ultimate cause of calcium malabsorption remains unknown.

Osteoporosis was first described in medical texts in the mid-1920s, and it became relatively easy to detect between 1920 and 1930 because X-rays started to be routinely used as a diagnostic tool during that period. In fact, X-rays were *over-used*, partly because they had a "new toy" aura and partly because no one yet knew the dangers inherent in radiation. The marvel of being able to visualize the inside of the body without having to cut into it made X-rays instantly popular—*too* popular.

Between 1930 and 1950 Americans dramatically increased their life span because of the burgeoning of new medical information, the advent of antibiotics, and the reduced death rate from infectious and communicable diseases. During this time the awareness of osteoporosis as a serious hazard to the elderly increased; and as old people become a significantly larger proportion of the population, the problem of osteoporosis will also increase. One estimate is that os-

---

*A collagen disease is a disease of the connective tissue that usually affects the entire body. There is some evidence now to show that these diseases may be caused by a genetic defect in the immune system. They are also referred to as autoimmune diseases.

teoporosis now costs Americans a billion dollars a year, but that seems low in light of the permanent crippling effects of the disease.

The economic burden of osteoporosis is enormous. Each year approximately 200,000 women suffer fractures that are directly attributable to the disease, and 40,000 of them die of fracture complications. In fact, 30 percent of all women and 17 percent of all men will suffer at least one hip fracture by age 90, and hip fractures result in a 12 percent decrease in life expectancy. They are a significant cause of death. In addition, 24 percent of all women and 5 percent of all men will suffer a Colles fracture.

It is likely that a survivor of a hip fracture will never walk again. A full 50 percent of those who break a hip will never be able to live independently, and a large proportion will require permanent nursing home care.

According to Joseph Melton and Laurence Riggs of the Mayo Foundation for Medical Education and Research in Rochester, Minnesota, "Elderly patients actually have a lower incidence of medically attended injuries each year than do young adults, but they are hospitalized more frequently and die as a result of the injury much more often. Although persons with reduced bone density may be subjected to severe trauma like anyone else, they are uniquely at risk for fractures sustained with moderate trauma of the sort that rarely results in fractures among young people. . . . The most common cause, by far, of fractures among elderly persons is a simple fall from a standing height or less. A third or more of all elderly individuals experience such a fall each year, and those age 65 or older count for about three quarters of the fatal falls recorded in the U.S. each year."[2]

Melton and Riggs emphasize that most falls occur indoors, and surprisingly, only eight percent occur because of people slipping on snow or ice. The fact that a simple fall from a standing height or less, which in people with normal bone density would produce nothing more than a surprised look,*

---

*A Colles fracture, however, is an exception. When a person of any age or bone strength falls on a hand outstretched to the side and rear in an effort to regain balance, he or she is likely to break a wrist.

can result in a break in an elderly person's hip or back attests to the extreme fragility of older bones.

Not all osteoporoses are created equal; that is, Laurence Riggs has identified four distinct types: age-related, senile, that associated with hyperparathyroidism (overactivity of the parathyroid gland), and that associated with impaired bone formation.

Age-related Osteoporosis

The cause of postmenopausal osteoporosis was first described in 1940, and as we have said, it affects far more females than males (the ratio is about 10:1). The most common clinical manifestation is a vertebra(e) fracture, but a Colles fracture is also common. Again, the cause is most likely subnormal calcium absorption or impaired metabolism of that mineral. "Nevertheless," says Riggs, "the menopause incompletely explains postmenopausal osteoporosis. All postmenopausal women are relatively estrogen-deficient, but osteoporosis develops in only some of them. Osteoporotic women could have a diminished production of sex steroid menopausally, [but] we could not confirm this finding. Thus, small differences in serum sex steroids between normal and osteoporotic postmenopausal women, even if present, probably do not play a major role in pathogenesis [the origin of a disease process]."[3]

In other words, lack of sex steroids alone cannot cause postmenopausal osteoporosis because, even though all women have diminished ovarian estrogen at menopause, not all menopausal women get osteoporosis.

Riggs goes on to say that science has been unable to prove that postmenopausal women with osteoporosis have a diminished responsiveness of estrogen-dependent tissue (such as the sexual and reproductive organs) to estrogen.

What, then, are the differences in postmenopausal women that make some of them more susceptible to osteoporosis than others? This is a major unanswered question and will require years of research.

Senile Osteoporosis

In people over age 75, senile osteoporosis is different from the postmenopausal type, says Riggs. The female to male ratio is only 2:1, and hip fracture is much more common than either broken wrist or back. "Only about 5% of postmenopausal women have fractures caused by osteoporosis before age 65 years, whereas by age 90 years, the cumulative incidence of fractures in the hip is 32% and in the vertebrae about 50%."[4]

What this means is that all fractures, but especially in the hip or back, are age-related; that is, the older a person is, the more likely he or she is to break something.

Riggs says that another characteristic of senile osteoporosis is that there is a relatively small decrease in bone density, and that occurs equally in the spongy and the dense bone. In postmenopausal osteoporosis, there is a disproportionately large decrease in spongy bone, which may account for the difference in fracture sites.

Why do bones age at different rates from other body tissues, and why is bone loss irreversible, whereas some other ravages of aging can be treated or even reversed? This is another major area for medical research.

Hyperparathyroidism

The parathyroid is a pea-sized endocrine gland located near, or even sometimes imbedded in, the thyroid gland in the neck. It secretes parathyroid hormone (PTH, sometimes called parathormone) that regulates the metabolism of calcium and phosphorus. Too little PTH causes overexcitability of the neuromuscular system, a decrease in blood calcium, and an increase in phosphorus. Other symptoms are cataracts, teeth defects, bone lesions, malformation of the hair and nails, and skin problems.

Too much PTH, hyperparathyroidism, causes a rise in blood calcium and a diminution in blood phosphorus. Calcium is removed from the bones, and they become fragile. There is also muscle weakness, poor muscle tone, and a generally sluggish functioning of the entire neuromuscular system.

When people age, they generally have an increased amount of PTH circulating in their blood, and this leads to a greater and greater imbalance between bone formation and bone resorption. Calcium absorption decreases with advancing age, especially after age 60; thus, we have osteoporosis associated with hyperparathyroidism, which Riggs thinks accounts for about 15 percent of the total number of cases of osteoporosis.

Impaired Bone Formation

Riggs also believes that a defect in bone formation may be a cause, but this is difficult to prove. He hypothesizes, however, that this defect prevents or limits the response of bone to sodium fluoride, which is a potent stimulator of bone formation. Possibly this is due to an intrinsic defect in the osteoblasts, or bone forming cells, or in the way they function. Then again, it may be caused by some impairment of the local control mechanisms (those in the bones themselves rather than in the circulating hormones or minerals) that regulate bone remodeling. Relatively few cases of osteoporosis arise from a defect in bone formation.

But whatever the cause and whatever the type, the end result of osteoporosis is the same: pain, crippling, permanent disability, economic disaster, and physical and psychological devastation.

Chapter Two

DIAGNOSIS AND TREATMENT

*O*steoporosis is difficult to diagnose except when it is obvious to even the most casual observer: when the osteoporotic person fractures a bone, especially the spine, wrist, or hip, and when the disease is clearly evident to either the naked eye or an ordinary X-ray machine. By then, however, the disease is far advanced, and there is little hope of significant improvement.

As with all diseases, osteoporosis should be diagnosed as early as possible in order to provide the most effective treatment. That treatment may correct damage before it becomes too severe, and it may prevent further diminution of bone mass.

Of all the noninvasive* diagnostic techniques described below, none is *absolutely* diagnostic of early osteoporosis. Thus, the goal of diagnosis and treatment is elusive. The diagnostic procedures measure either total bone mass or total bone calcium. The reason they do not produce a definitive diagnosis is because although the leading cause of fractures in postmenopausal women and elderly people in general is diminished mineralized bone, this is not the only cause. We shall describe some of the other causes later in the chapter.

---

*Noninvasive means that no instrument or other device enters the body. Examples of invasive procedures are surgery, blood tests, biopsy, a rectal or pelvic examination, spinal tap, or even just taking the temperature.

Because 98 to 99 percent of total body calcium (TBC) is in the skeleton, the more calcium you have in your bones, the stronger they are. The latter can be calculated by measuring TBC by a variety of noninvasive techniques.

Some of the diagnostic techniques described below are more accurate than others, and some are easier to do than others. In general, the more accurate the test, the more sophisticated it is, and the equipment and technical expertise are at the forefront of high technology. This almost ensures that the procedure will be expensive.

Some of the tests, such as neutron activation analysis (NAA), are so new that they are still mostly experimental and are available at only a few medical centers. While they are not now practical as diagnostic tools, we list them here because experimental medical techniques have a habit of quickly becoming routine. The line between science fiction and medical reality has blurred somewhat lately, and some of the tests for osteoporosis involve radiation and radiographic emissions. The reader may be reminded of *Star Trek*® when Dr. Bones would pass a futuristic wand over one of the Starship *Enterprise*'s crew members, look at some flashing lights and numbers on a computer, and then come up with a diagnosis. The diagnostic "wands" of X-ray departments in medical centers are huge, very expensive and cumbersome machines, but the principle of noninvasive diagnosis is no longer a futuristic fantasy. The techniques used to diagnose osteoporosis are:

• X-ray. This is the oldest, least accurate, and least sensitive diagnostic tool. Its lack of sensitivity results from the fact that as much as 40 percent of TBC can be lost before it is detectable on X-ray, and by that time the disease is far advanced. There is also great variability in both exposure factors and the interpretation of films. This kind of inappropriate individuality lowers diagnostic accuracy. However, ordinary X-ray is still the way most people's osteoporosis is diagnosed.

• Long bone weight. The weight of long bones (those in the arms and legs) correlates with total skeletal weight. Therefore, weighing long bones (by weighing the entire limb and subtracting nonbone tissue weight) can be somewhat predictive of the weight of bones elsewhere in the skeleton. However, absolute accuracy is never possible because all diseased bone does not degenerate at the same rate; while weighing long bones is fairly accurate (but unnecessary) when the person is healthy, it is less so in the presence of osteoporosis. If osteoporosis is suspected, it is much better to weigh the entire skeleton, although this is more difficult.

• The Norland-Cameron Bone Mineral Analyzer. This device measures bone density at the end of the radius (one of the two long bones between the elbow and the wrist) of the nondominant hand, that is, the left hand of a right-handed person and vice versa. The analyzer measures both cortical (dense) and trabecular (spongy) bone.

• Radiogrammetry. This is the measurement of a metacarpal bone's cortical thickness. A metacarpal is one of the five bones in the hand between the wrist and the fingers. The technique can calculate the amount of cortical bone, but it cannot measure the amount of absolute bone. It is precise about small changes in bone thickness but not about changes in bone mineral. Because it is a readily available technique, it is used often and is helpful in estimating relative changes in bone.

• CAT scan. Computerized axial tomography (also known as a CT scan or CAT) measures the density of trabecular bone in the vertebrae and elsewhere. A CAT scan is a complex system of thousands of high-speed X-rays taken at various tissue level penetrations. The X-rays are then collated by computer to provide a precise computer picture of the tissue scanned. The advantage of the CAT scan over an ordinary X-ray is that it "slices" the tissue and takes pictures from all 360-degree angles. Thus, the entire bone, not just the surface, can be visualized.

• Photon absorptiometry. Absorptiometry is a method of instrumental analysis in which the absorption (or absence of absorption) of selected electromagnetic radiation is a qualitative and quantitative indication of the chemical composition of the tissue under examination, in this case bone. The type of radiation used ranges from radio and microwave through infrared, visible, and ultraviolet radiation to X-rays and gamma rays.

A photon is a quotient of electromagnetic radiation; photon absorptiometry is a process by which a beam of electromagnetic energy is used to scan bones. If a single beam is used, it can scan only peripheral bones (those closest to the surface of the body), which are composed primarily of cortical bone. If a dual beam is used, total body mineral and mass can be measured. This means that both cortical and trabecular bone can be scanned, and the measurement correlates with the strength of the vertebral column, or spine.

Photon absorptiometry is a highly precise measurement of the bones in the path of the scanning electromagnetic beam because the radioactive iodides given to the person absorb the beam and then transmit measurable radiation. The presence of certain skeletal minerals is proportional to changes in electromagnetic beam intensity and thus is a measure of the presence and extent of osteoporosis. Photon absorptiometry is a highly sophisticated diagnostic tool that requires skilled technicians. This means that not only is it not available everywhere but that it is quite expensive.

• Total body neutron activation analysis (NAA). This procedure measures TBC. A person is irradiated by a process that converts stable calcium to radioactive calcium which emits gamma rays with a half-life of 8.8 minutes. This extremely short half-life means that the body's calcium reverts to normal in a short time.

The gamma rays are measured for the presence and amount of radioactive calcium which is then compared to a standard for normal people. This gives an index of the TBC and is precise to within two percent.

The purpose of NAA is to detect the presence of osteopenia, a diminution of mineralized bone, to quantify the severity of the osteopenia, and to measure the response to treatment.

There are drawbacks to NAA: Even when it becomes routine, it will still be almost prohibitively expensive. Moreover, though it is possible to assess precisely the extent of osteopenia, it is difficult to determine the *significance* of bone mineral loss because there is so wide a variety of bone mass in normal people of similar size. Therefore, determining when a loss of mineralized bone becomes truly pathologic and when it is acceptable and/or safe becomes an educated guessing game.

• Bone biopsy. This is an invasive procedure in which a

small plug of bone is withdrawn, usually from the top of the flat, flaring hip bone, the iliac crest. The crest is easily accessible, and a sample taken from it will include both cortical and trabecular bone.

There's no escaping the fact that a bone biopsy hurts. It's not agonizing, however, and the pain lasts only a short time—as long as the procedure lasts. Although skin, muscle, and periosteum (the tough membrane or sheath covering bone) can be anesthetized, bone cannot, and when the trocar, the sharp pointed instrument with a serrated edge, pierces the bone, it hurts. As soon as the trocar is removed, however, the pain is relieved, although the person who has had a bone biopsy feels sore and bruised for a day or so. A pathologist then examines the bone sample under a microscope, giving it various bone mineral content tests, and notes the presence and activity of osteoblasts and osteoclasts.

All the diagnostic tests described above are difficult and expensive to some extent, although some are simpler than others, and with the exception of X-ray, the vast majority of orthopedic physicians (called orthopods) do not use them to diagnose osteoporosis. Rather, they find the disease by a process called differential diagnosis, that is, by taking a series of symptoms and risk factors into account and then ruling out other diseases that have similar symptoms. When other possibilities have been eliminated (usually because they are easier to diagnose), osteoporosis is left.

Differential diagnosis is a standard part of the medical repertoire. For example, if a person complains of coughing, chest pain, shortness of breath, and fever, the doctor is faced with several choices of illness, such as pneumonia, tuberculosis, lung cancer, and a severe chest cold. He or she performs a series of diagnostic tests and asks the patient questions to determine the likelihood of this, that, or the other disease. Lung cancer can be ruled out, for example, by a biopsy of lung tissue, and tuberculosis is discarded if the patient's sputum has no trace of the *tubercle bacillus*.

Differential diagnosis can rule out other bone diseases. According to C. Conrad Johnston and Solomon Epstein, osteomalacia (the softening of bones due to decreased mineralization resulting mostly from a Vitamin D deficiency) is the other major diagnostic possibility. "Patients with osteomalacia frequently complain of more persistent pain but do not have the episodes of acute pain associated with vertebral collapse fracture [as in osteoporosis]."[1]

Other blood tests can eliminate other diseases, and most doctors make a diagnosis of osteoporosis based on observation, close questioning of the patient, microscopic examination of the blood and urine, and perhaps some X-rays.

No "fancy" tests are involved. The patient doesn't go near a CAT scanner and is not subjected to electromagnetic radiation. This is not to say that the more sophisticated tests are not valuable; indeed they are. It *is* to say, rather, that most physicians don't have access to such advanced technology; many don't know what's available and many, if they did know, would advise against it because of the expense. Moreover, many patients don't see orthopods. They are diagnosed by their general practitioner, or even sometimes by a gynecologist, who may be less likely to know about advanced diagnostic techniques for osteoporosis. So most times the doctor diagnoses the disease with his or her eyes, ears, and brain.

The other diseases that must be ruled out because they cause some of the same symptoms as osteoporosis are:

• "Hyperthyroidism," according to Johnston and Epstein, "is associated with accelerated bone loss that may result in fractures. It can generally be easily diagnosed from the clinical [those observable to the physician] features and with the use of proper laboratory studies. However, [it] is more common in the aging population among whom osteoporosis also occurs. Thus a high index of suspicion must be maintained."[2]

• Hyperparathyroidism* is also associated with accelerated bone loss and a high incidence of vertebral fracture. Calcium levels in the blood can distinguish it from osteoporosis.

• Glucocorticoid excess. A corticoid is a hormone secreted by one of the adrenal glands, located just above each kidney, and a glucocorticoid is one that stimulates glucose

---

*The parathyroid gland, located in the neck near the thyroid, controls metabolism of calcium and phosphorus.

(sugar) production and thus raises the blood sugar level. An excessive amount of glucocorticoids leads to bone loss and vertebral fractures. A careful monitoring of blood sugar levels should distinguish it from osteoporosis.

• Cancer that has spread to the spine from elsewhere in the body can cause vertebral fractures. Sometimes, particularly in the elderly, the original cancer has not been diagnosed; that is, the person does not know that he or she has cancer. However, since the vertebrae break in a unique way in metastatic cancer, that should alert the physician. A bone biopsy will provide a definitive diagnosis of cancer.

One of the most important factors in diagnosing disease is the statistical likelihood of one's having a particular disease. But just because someone is at high risk for a disease doesn't mean that he or she will get it. A competent physician will consider the odds when making a diagnosis. If a severely malnourished alcoholic comes to the doctor coughing, tuberculosis is a strong possibility because alcoholics are at particularly high risk for TB. This is only a clue, however, and the physician will still have to look for the *tubercle bacillus* in the person's sputum in order to confirm the diagnosis.

Risk factors for osteoporosis include the following:

• Alcoholism is one of the strongest risks for osteoporosis. It is unclear why alcoholics should be at such high risk, but some scientists speculate that they tend to have poor calcium absorption, although they are not at particularly high risk for osteomalacia.

• Diabetes mellitus

• Intestinal bypass surgery, done sometimes to remove a malignancy and sometimes to combat severe obesity,* decreases the absorption of all nutrients, including calcium and Vitamin D.

• Where you live. Osteoporosis is more prevalent in temperate zones than in the tropics. This may have something to do with the higher ultraviolet radiation levels in the tropics which stimulate absorption of Vitamin D.

_____

*This is a highly controversial and dangerous procedure.

• Race. Osteoporosis occurs more among whites than nonwhites. Blacks have substantially greater bone density than whites, which may or may not be a genetic predisposition; it also may be a result of living in more tropical climates than whites.

• Low body weight. Thin women with a light skeletal frame are at higher risk of osteoporosis than those who are bigger.

• A family history of osteoporosis

• Smaller than average muscle mass in proportion to bone

• Lack of exercise or a sedentary life style

• Low calcium intake

• Early menopause or oophorectomy (surgical removal of the ovaries)

• Cigarette smoking

• Greater than normal consumption of protein, fiber, and caffeine. Vegetarians have a lower than average risk of osteoporosis.

• Low body fat. Obese women rarely develop osteoporosis because estrogen is stored in subcutaneous fat (fat stored beneath the skin) and continues to be released long after menopause. Moreover, androgen, a male hormone, is converted to estrogen by adipose (fatty) tissue after menopause.*

• Childlessness. Estrogen production increases markedly during pregnancy, and although women aren't permanently pregnant, of course, some scientists theorize that the temporary increase in estrogen production has a permanent positive effect on bone by stimulating the production of calcitonin and the activation of Vitamin D. However, no one knows exactly why bearing children lowers the risk of osteoporosis.

• Taking drugs such as corticosteroids, phenobarbital, aluminum-containing antacids (such as Gelusil and Maalox), some diuretics, and thyroxin

---

*Obesity is one of the best preventions against osteoporosis, but at the same time it creates a wide variety of other health hazards, most particularly cardiovascular disease. This creates a conflict for women who want to prevent both of these extremely debilitating conditions.

• Drinking nonfluoridated water

• Oral contraceptives seem to have an inhibitory effect on osteoporosis, although no one knows why. The estrogen in the pills may have the same kind of positive influence on bone that pregnancy does.

Before 1925 there was absolutely no treatment for osteoporosis. Now the treatment is only minimally effective.

During the period between the two world wars, research was begun to study the effect of estrogen on bone. It is now clear that there is a significant relationship between the amount of circulating and stored estrogen and the amount of bone tissue. Moreover, it is also clear that estrogen replacement therapy (ERT) after menopause can retard the development of osteoporosis and *may* even contribute to the formation of new bone. ERT is fully discussed in Chapter 3.

Beginning in about 1935, scientists developed an interest in parathyroid hormone (PTH) and its role in stimulating osteoclasts to resorb bone and rob it of calcium. That role has since been well established.

At about the same time, researchers began human studies in which they gave people various amounts of dietary calcium, phosphorus, magnesium, Vitamin D, and other substances to determine the effect on bone. Says Harold M. Frost, "By 1980 the outcome of those numerous efforts could be distilled into one sentence: all failed to restore the bone tissue volume deficit of senile osteoporosis, but somehow supplementary dietary calcium seemed to retard future bone loss as long as patients took it."[3]

Further research has proved that trabecular or spongy bone volume can be increased after the osteoporotic process has begun, and perhaps even more important, bone loss can be avoided to a great extent if prevention is begun early, that is, if calcium intake is increased long before the onset of middle age.

It is believed that one of the best ways to increase the amount of trabecular bone is with concurrent, continuous administration of supplemental calcium, fluoride, and Vitamin D. This combination therapy, although known to be effective, is still under investigation to determine, according to Frost, ". . . (1) whether or not the treatment can add new bone without limit to any desired degree, (2) if that bone remains permanently in place after cessation of therapy, (3) if similar changes occur in compact [cortical or dense] bone, and (4) if, in fact, the treated patients subsequently have less disability than they would have had if untreated. Thus, control groups, cortical bone studies, and an accurate description of the natural course of untreated osteoporosis will prove necessary. Longer observation must reveal whether or not short- or long-term adverse effects result from the treatment. Finally, further work must determine optimal doses, choice of agents [drugs], and schedules for their administration."[4]

There is now no doubt, though, that calcium alone has a significant effect on bone, and it is especially effective in women who are also taking replacement estrogen (or who still have enough of their own). But even without the extra estrogen, calcium is beneficial. Robert R. Recker says, "Recently longitudinal studies [in which research subjects are observed over a long period of time] of patients with deliberately elevated calcium intakes have shown that high intakes of about 1.5 gm [1500 mg] of calcium per day will inhibit age-related bone loss in white women past menopause when observed for two years."[5]

Other studies have shown that people who have had a relatively high lifelong daily intake of calcium (1000 mg or more per day) have a lower incidence of fracture than those who take less calcium. Further, when calcium is deliberately reduced, bone loss is accelerated.

Recker concludes, "It seems clear, then, that higher calcium intakes do help preserve the skeleton in postmenopausal women and a total intake of about 1.5 gm per day is convenient and effective. The self-selected diet can be supplemented with calcium carbonate, calcium lactate, or one of the other commercial preparations containing calcium. It should be noted that calcium supplements alone have not been shown to *increase* bone mass, and in the studies that directly compared the effect of calcium supplements with that of estrogens, the estrogens came out slightly better."[6]

Calcium supplements are available in any drugstore or supermarket without a prescription. Most of the tablets do not contain pure calcium, and many are combined with other elements. Some have Vitamin D to help your body absorb the calcium. The amount of pure (or elemental) calcium varies widely from product to product and from one chemical preparation to another, and the only way to tell how much actual pure calcium is in each tablet is to *read the label*.

Many drug companies have jumped on the calcium-for-menopausal-women bandwagon, and it's almost impossible to pick up a women's magazine these days without seeing several full-page advertisements for this or that brand of calcium supplement. The name of the preparation is far less important than the amount of pure calcium in each tablet, and a heavily advertised national brand is no better than a house brand or private label calcium supplement. See the chart at the end of the chapter for a representative sample of calcium supplement prices.

A house brand or private label is that of a particular store or chain of stores. Most large chains of drugstores and supermarkets buy drugs such as aspirin, vitamins, antacids, and laxatives in enormous quantities from pharmaceutical companies and affix their own labels. The stores don't advertise these products and don't wrap them in fancy packages. The bottles simply sit quietly on the shelf—at significantly lower prices than their nationally advertised counterparts. It would be a good idea to spend 15 minutes or so studying the wide variety of bottles of calcium supplements (with a calculator if necessary) before settling on a brand. The more carefully one decides at the beginning, the better shape one's bones—and wallet—will be in.

There is some controversy about the effectiveness of calcium supplements on bone that is so severely osteoporotic that it is excessively fragile. Such porous bone tends to absorb calcium slowly, but even so, additional calcium might be beneficial because it tends to minimize further bone loss. There is almost no risk of side effects as a result of high doses of calcium. But it is wise to remember that bone loss is almost always worse than it appears on X-ray; therefore, the good that extra calcium can do far outweighs whatever minimal risk there is. In other words, it's never too late to start taking calcium supplements.

There have been no reported untoward effects when

healthy menopausal women take calcium supplements, but most physicians recommend monitoring blood and urine calcium levels. If the level of circulating calcium is too high, the dose can be lowered. Your blood pressure should also be checked at least every six months.

Those who take the supplementary calcium should be aware that although it *can* increase bone volume, it is *not* a cure for osteoporosis because the disease is not specifically a result of calcium deficiency, as, for example, scurvy is specifically caused by a deficiency of Vitamin C. Although too little calcium is probably a prime cause of fractures in old age, it is not the only one. Genetic make-up, bone tissue quality, physical activity, hormonal influences, and the propensity to fall are other factors.

For example, black women in the United States have a lower lifelong calcium intake than do white women, yet they have a much lower incidence of postmenopausal osteoporosis and fractures. Black African women have both lower calcium intake and lower bone mass than white women, yet they suffer fewer fractures. In both these cases, genetics and physical activity probably play a more significant role in later-life osteoporosis than does calcium intake.

The role of fluoride supplements in treating osteoporosis is still unclear. There is some evidence that it stimulates the production of new bone, but the safety of high doses of fluoride has not yet been established.

The use of Vitamin D, alone or in combination with calcium and/or fluoride, has been somewhat successful. It is not clear whether Vitamin D acts directly on osteoblasts, stimulating them to produce more bone, or whether it acts indirectly by raising calcium concentrations. The meaning of too little Vitamin D is also unclear; that is, is the problem the amount of circulating Vitamin D, or is there a malfunction in the absorption of the vitamin?

Recker concludes: "Few would argue with the idea that vitamin D deficiency should be avoided if possible in all people, particularly in elderly postmenopausal women whose dietary intake and exposure to sun may be marginal. Even mild deficiency will depress calcium absorption and cause negative calcium (bone) balance. The bone loss is probably largely reversible if the deficiency is short term.

However, very long-term mild vitamin D deficiency may result in irreversible bone loss such as that seen in some patients many years after gastric or bowel surgery. Adequate levels of vitamin D should be guaranteed both in healthy postmenopausal women and those with osteoporosis by administration of at least 400 units daily in the form of multivitamins or by exposure to a sun lamp for about 15 minutes daily."*[7]

Megadoses of Vitamin D (some people take as much as 5000 to 50,000 units a day) will not stimulate new bone formation or prevent fractures, even when taken in combination with calcium. There is also evidence that too much Vitamin D will cause headaches, nausea, dizziness, blurred vision, excessive fatigue, and kidney and nervous system damage.

Most multivitamin tablets available in drugstores and supermarkets without a prescription contain 400 to 500 units of Vitamin D: an adequate daily dose. An alternative to a multivitamin, if the diet is lacking in Vitamin D, is Vitamin D–enhanced calcium supplements.

It may or may not be possible to augment bone mass later in life, but almost all research on the treatment of osteoporosis is directed toward that effort. There are three times in one's life when there is a rapid and significant increase in bone volume, only one of which may have significance for osteoporosis research: adolescence, pregnancy, and during periods of heavy physical exertion. It is with the last that we are most concerned. According to Recker, "It is now well known that physical activity and mechanical stress influence bone mass. Bone is rapidly lost during bed rest, weightlessness,** or paralysis, and bone mass is positively

---

*Using a sun lamp has become highly controversial because of the connection between ultraviolet rays and skin cancer.
**One of the most interesting medical observations to come out of the early space program was the amount of bone tissue the astronauts lost even on very short space flights. The sedentary life in orbit was a particularly drastic change for the astronauts who had been accustomed to regular strenuous physical exercise.

correlated with muscle mass. The most important mechanical stress seems to be weight-bearing in the upright posture. However, it has been difficult to demonstrate that consciously increasing physical activity results in a further increase in bone mass. It now seems clear that heavy physical exertion, especially in the adolescent years, results in a measurable increase in bone mass; the adolescent phase of expanding bone mass may itself be augmented by heavy exertion. Consciously increasing physical activity among adults may not be a practical way of augmenting bone mass, since short-term experiments with moderate increases in exertion have not been successful and investigators have had to examine highly trained athletes or marathon runners in order to find effects.

"On the other hand, increased physical activity may protect against fractures without increasing bone mass."[8]

This may be due to the development of greater muscle mass which protects bones, or there may be another, as yet undiscovered, cause.

It appears, then, that moderate physical activity is both desirable and practical,* but heavy exertion is not only impractical for older people, it will not do much good in terms of augmenting bone mass or preventing fractures. In other words, older people should not begin an exercise program that rivals an Army boot camp, nor is it necessary to spend money on expensive and elaborate work-out equipment. It's best to have been exercising for one's entire life, but even if one has been completely sedentary up until middle age, there is still benefit in starting—slowly and carefully—a regimen of moderate exercise.

Although we will discuss the treatment of fractures in a separate chapter, there are some general treatment considerations that apply to all people with osteoporosis, especially how to deal with pain.

A vertebral fracture, called a compression fracture, usually results from some innocuous activity that would have no effect on a person without osteoporosis: bending down to

---

*See the chapter on exercise for descriptions of the most beneficial moderate exercises.

pick up the cat, lifting something not particularly heavy, or even getting out of a deep armchair. People with osteoporosis are particularly vulnerable to minor accidents, such as being jerked suddenly when a car in which they are riding comes to a screeching panic stop* or falling from as low as standing height. Such ordinary events that would not faze a healthy person can break an osteoporotic vertebra and cause excruciating pain. The break is most often in the middle of the back from about mid-chest to waist level.

The person who breaks a vertebra is usually plunged into severe and immediate pain, although in rare instances the pain may not gear up to full force for a day or two. Physical activity, even coughing, laughing, or deep breathing, makes the pain worse; immobility relieves it somewhat. People with vertebral fractures are highly reluctant to move.

Compression fractures heal well with almost no medical treatment. The only thing the person must do is to lie flat in bed (not necessarily on the back but not in a sitting or reclining position) for seven to ten days until the worst of the acute pain has passed. After that, the person can sit up for increasingly longer periods of time (but starting with very short periods; for example, ten minutes) while wearing a heavy canvas back brace. Then he or she can begin walking at frequent but short intervals, lengthening them gradually until recovery is complete. This takes varying amounts of time, depending on the person's general strength, physical condition, and how well he or she follows the prescribed program, but three or four months is average.

After the acute phase has passed, the worst problem for most people is the tedium of enforced rest and inactivity. One's life is generally disrupted for the entire time the fracture is healing. The only kind of work one can do is that which involves only the brain and perhaps the telephone or a dictating machine. There's no going into the office or back to the factory. There's no housecleaning or running out to do errands. Life becomes circumscribed and narrow, and this is difficult for most people.

---

*A seat belt and shoulder harness may prevent an accident of this type.

Hospitalization is not medically necessary beyond the first day or so, but bed rest is *mandatory*. In situations where the person with a broken back has family (or servants) to fetch and carry (food, bedpan, bath water, books, the television set—*everything* the patient wants and needs), there may be little problem other than boredom. However, almost no one is that lucky, especially women who live alone or have husbands who must go to work every day. They will have to make other arrangements for care. Hiring an aide for 24-hour care is prohibitively expensive for everyone except the very few. General hospitals will not keep patients who do not require acute medical treatment because insurance companies will not pay for "custodial" care. There is now no such thing as languishing in a hospital bed for months with treatment requirements no more sophisticated than an order for bed rest with gradually increasing activity and an occasional laxative or enema.

There may be only one choice left: a nursing home. This is an unpleasant, even frightening, prospect because, although there are a few well-run, caring, professional nursing homes (most of which are run by religious groups), most are simply dumping grounds for the elderly and infirm who have nowhere else to go, no one to take care of them, and not enough money to pay for home care or a good nursing home.

The one bright spot in this gloomy picture is that the situation is not permanent; the fracture will heal, and the person can look forward to being discharged. Moreover, if the person confined to a nursing home can demand the prescribed schedule of rest and activity, or if there is a friend or relative who is willing to supervise the care and make certain that orders are carried out, being "sentenced" to a nursing home need not be a hopeless prospect.

Compression fractures not only heal completely, but the broken vertebra is usually stronger than it was before and stronger than the others in the spine. However, if the regimen of rest and activity is not adhered to while the vertebra is healing, it will collapse further, possibly leading to a severe and permanent deformity known as kyphosis, or "dowager's hump," the lump-like curvature of the spine that is so common in older women.

The acute pain of a vertebral fracture passes in two weeks

or so, but it is often supplanted by chronic low back pain, possibly because the person places increased stress on other parts of the spine to compensate for the pain of the fracture. Lying horizontally will almost always relieve the pain, but some people are unwilling to spend long hours lying flat. They usually pay for this with an exceptionally long recuperation period in which they generally feel well in the morning but end up in severe pain as the day wears on. Sometimes the pain is so severe that it is not relieved by lying down.

Frost says that pain medication is not the answer to this problem. "Patients going through this phase should not receive analgesics for their pain. By that pain, nature signals the need for intermittent horizontal rest, which fortunately rarely fails to provide desired relief. I see a number of such patients annually whom other physicians have treated with analgesics and some type of back support but not with intermittent horizontal rest. Such patients can remain uncomfortable literally for years until they go on an intermittent rest regimen for two to four months."[9]

In about five percent of all osteoporosis patients this regimen of intermittent horizontal rest doesn't help, and they have chronic bone pain. Some have aching pain along most of the spine, sometimes even over the ribs, that becomes worse when they stand erect. In addition, the pelvis, knees, and ankles can ache. The reason for the pain remains a mystery, but that is of little consolation to the person who is near tears whenever he or she stands or walks. Sometimes there are personality changes because the pain becomes the central focus of existence. When things get this far out of control, professional help is necessary—perhaps from one of the many pain control clinics that have been established in medical centers across the country.

Horizontal rest will occasionally help a little, but it doesn't entirely relieve the pain. Mild analgesics such as aspirin, acetaminophen (Tylenol), or a combination of aspirin, phenacetin, and caffeine (APC) are only minimally effective, and anything stronger, such as a narcotic, is not advisable because of the potential for dependence. Frost says that the bone pain of osteoporosis is usually self-limiting; that is, it disappears spontaneously within a few years—ordinarily not more than five—and he recommends time, patience, and lots of horizontal rest.

An experimental process may some day be applied to the treatment of osteoporosis: making new bone from old. The technique is dramatic, almost miraculous in a way, and has a science fiction aura about it.

Bone taken from human or animal cadavers is cut into small chips and pulverized into granules. It is then bathed in a solution of hydrochloric acid, alcohol, and ether to remove the calcium, phosphorus, and other minerals. The granules are then washed, heated, and mixed with water to form a paste called demineralized bone matrix (DBM).

This paste is surgically implanted in the body and for reasons not yet understood, it transforms adjacent cells into osteoblasts which begin to manufacture first cartilage and then bone. The process takes several months, but the bone is every bit as real as that produced without DBM.

The resorption rate is low, and although the long-term effects remain to be seen, the bone has been used successfully for five years. A child in Boston, in fact, had his entire skull replaced by this process and is doing well.

DBM may one day be used in place of bone grafts and to join the two edges of a fractured bone for faster and stronger healing. The latter would be especially beneficial for osteoporosis sufferers whose fractures take especially long to mend. Compressed vertebrae might be fused with DBM, thereby preventing future compression fractures, and it might be used to completely replace destroyed bone. When the gene that is responsible for the transformation of other cells into osteoblasts is cloned, the commercial possibilities of DBM can be realized, and it will be in common use.

Treatment for osteoporosis is "iffy" at best, and even though supplemental calcium can increase bone volume and mass, there is no cure for the disease. The best course of action remains prevention and the diminution of risk wherever possible. Although one can't change one's race or basic skeletal structure, there *are* things to be done to minimize the risk of osteoporosis:

- Increase calcium intake *before* menopause to about 1000 mg a day.
- Eat less protein, especially the complete proteins found in meat.
- Make certain your water supply is fluoridated.
- Drink less alcohol.
- Stop smoking.
- Begin a program of moderate regular exercise.

The chart that follows shows the wide variation in calcium supplement prices. The price sample was taken in Montgomery County, Maryland, just outside Washington, D.C., on December 10, 1984. Although the range of prices may be higher in Washington than in some parts of the country, the variation is probably representative.

The most important part of the label on a bottle of calcium supplement is the amount of *pure* (elemental) calcium in each tablet. Those brands that contain calcium bound with another chemical (for instance calcium carbonate) are not necessarily all pure calcium. However, the actual amount of the mineral is always somewhere on the label, usually in small print. It's essential to know precisely how much calcium one is getting.

Also, some brands label the amount by the recommended daily dose; that is, the label indicates the amount of calcium in two, three, or four tablets, and the consumer must do some arithmetic to determine the dose of elemental calcium in *each* tablet.

Some companies manufacture the supplement in two different doses, packaged in boxes or bottles of the same size. However, the number of tablets in different bottles may vary. For example, Os Cal 250 and Os Cal 500 vary significantly in the number of tablets and dose, but the price per 1000 mg of calcium is almost the same. Therefore, it pays to read the label and do some arithmetic.

The stores chosen for the sample represent a cross section of the places where people shop for drugs. Not all the stores carried the same brands, and there are surely brands of calcium supplements not represented here.

Store No. 1 is a branch of People's, a large chain of drugstores in the Washington-Baltimore area.

Store No. 2 is a branch of Safeway, the largest supermarket chain in the country.

Store No. 3 is a branch of Dart Drug, a large local chain of discount drugstores.

Store No. 4 is a branch of Giant Foods, the largest chain of supermarkets in the Baltimore-Washington-Richmond area.

Store No. 5 is Bradley Care Drug, an independent drugstore in a middle class neighborhood.

Store No. 6 is Glen Echo Drugstore, an independent store in a fairly affluent area.

CALCIUM SUPPLEMENT PRICE COMPARISONS

Brand Name	Form of Calcium Preparation	Amount of Calcium (in mg) Per Tablet	Vitamin D (in units)	Other Elements	# Tablets in Bottle	Store #1 Price per Bottle	Price per 1000 mg Calcium
BioCal Chewable	carbonate	250	—	—	75	7.49	40¢
BioCal Chewable	carbonate	500	—	—	75	7.49	20¢
Calcet	gluconate lactate carbonate	240 240 240	100	—	100	7.99	11¢
Caltrate 600 (red box)	carbonate	600	125	—	60	6.79	18¢
Caltrate 600 (blue box)	carbonate	600	—	—	60	6.79	18¢
People's	carbonate	600	—	—	60	4.99	14¢
OsCal 250	oyster shell carbonate	250	125	—	100	7.09	28¢
OsCal 500	oyster shell carbonate	500	—	—	60	8.59	29¢
Nature Made	oyster shell	250	125	—	100	NS	
Safeway	dicalcium phosphate	270	400	phosphorus 170 mg	100	NS	
Safeway Dolomite	not indicated on label	500	—	magnesium 255 mg	250	NS	
Dart	carbonate	500	—	—	60	NS	
Lilly	carbonate	260	—	—	100	NS	
Abbot DICAL-D	phosphate	500	133	—	100	NS	
Giant	oyster shell	250	125	—	100	NS	
Giant Dolomite	oyster shell	130	—	magnesium 78 mg	250	NS	
Hudson	oyster shell	500	—	—	60	NS	

Store #2 Price per Bottle	Price per 1000 mg Calcium	Store #3 Price per Bottle	Price per 1000 mg Calcium	Store #4 Price per Bottle	Price per 1000 mg Calcium	Store #5 Price per Bottle	Price per 1000 mg Calcium	Store #6 Price per Bottle	Price per 1000 mg Calcium
Not Sold (NS)		6.29	30¢	7.59	40¢	8.14	43¢	8.15	43¢
NS		6.29	17¢	6.49	17¢	NS		NS	
NS		NS		NS		NS		NS	
NS		6.39	17¢	NS		7.95	22¢	NS	
4.99	14¢	6.39	17¢	6.39	17¢	7.95	20¢	NS	
NS		NS		NS		NS		NS	
6.88	28¢	7.59	30¢	6.88	28¢	8.14	33¢	8.15	33¢
7.59	25¢	9.59	32¢	7.59	25¢	9.57	32¢	9.57	32¢
2.99	12¢	NS		NS		NS		NS	
1.99	7¢	NS		NS		NS		NS	
3.19	3¢	NS		NS		NS		NS	
NS		4.79	16¢	NS		NS		NS	
NS		6.59	25¢	NS		NS		NS	
NS		7.89	16¢	NS		NS		NS	
NS		NS		2.42	10¢	NS		NS	
NS		NS		2.15	7¢	NS		NS	
NS		NS		NS		3.99	13¢	3.99	13¢

(continued on pages 46 and 47)

Brand Name	Form of Calcium Preparation	Amount of Calcium (in mg) Per Tablet	Vitamin D (in units)	Other Elements	# Tablets in Bottle	Store #1 Price per Bottle	Price per 1000 mg Calcium
Hudson Concentrate	carbonate	600	—	—	60	NS	
Lilly Chewable	gluconate	47	—	—	100	NS	
CalSup	carbonate	300	—	—	100	NS	
Nature's Bounty	oyster shell	375	200	—	100	NS	
Hudson	lactate	84.5	—	—	200	NS	
Hudson Natural	oyster shell	325	200	—	100	NS	

Store #2 Price per Bottle / Price per 1000 mg Calcium	Store #3 Price per Bottle / Price per 1000 mg Calcium	Store #4 Price per Bottle / Price per 1000 mg Calcium	Store #5 Price per Bottle / Price per 1000 mg Calcium	Store #6 Price per Bottle / Price per 1000 mg Calcium
NS	NS	NS	3.99 / 11¢	3.99 / 11¢
NS	NS	NS	7.68 / $1.63	NS
NS	NS	NS	8.71 / 30¢	8.72 / 30¢
NS	NS	NS	3.25 / 9¢	NS
NS	NS	NS	NS	4.49 / 26¢
NS	NS	NS	NS	3.19 / 10¢

Chapter Three

ESTROGEN REPLACEMENT THERAPY (ERT)

*T*he decision to take replacement estrogens should be yours alone. Your gynecologist cannot and should not decide for you, although you have to depend on him or her to give you the facts necessary to make the decision.

But if your doctor doesn't provide the facts, they are not easy to come by. Most well-educated and medically astute women don't read medical journal articles. Even if you had the time and inclination, you wouldn't have the background to decipher the medical jargon and get to the kernel of necessary information. The public press may not be much more help. As Dr. John Berryman, an obstetrician and gynecologist in private practice in Washington, D.C., and Assistant Clinical Professor of Obstetrics and Gynecology at George Washington University Medical School, says, "Good news doesn't get into print. Only the dramatic bad news makes it into the papers."

He was talking about the significant progress made in replacement estrogens in the past decade, most specifically about the amount of estrogen and progestogen contained in the pills, which has changed drastically. This fact has been underreported, and in some cases ignored, by the press.

Replacement estrogens did get some justified bad press in the mid to late 1970s, but the pills that are being marketed now are vastly different from the ones sold then. Many women are still leery of them, though. The question is, why?

"They're afraid of them," says Berryman, "because of the press. All the studies that were reported in the press were done on a very different pill [a much higher dose of estrogen], and I have a hard time getting that across. Look, would you call a 1928 Essex the same as a brand new Cadillac? It's the same with pills that contain estrogen."

But if the public press, especially daily newspapers, provides a mostly one-sided view of replacement estrogens (when it bothers to report it at all) and generally ignores the good news, which isn't nearly so dramatic, what are you to do? Most of us don't have the background necessary to read original medical research, so how *will* you get the facts necessary to make a wise decision?

There are two major ways, both equally important. The first is to choose a gynecologist who is interested in the science as well as the art (and business) of medicine. Finding one is not difficult if you are willing to "test" the doctor to see if he or she appears competent and interested. There are several ways to do this:

• Find out if he or she is board certified in obstetrics and gynecology. This means that the physician has had postgraduate medical education and training in gynecology, has done a three- to four-year residency in the specialty, and has passed an examination at the end of that time. The training program and examination are administered by the American College of Obstetricians and Gynecologists (ACOG), and the doctor should have a certificate hanging prominently in his office. If the certificate isn't there, ask if he or she is board certified. If the answer is no—or worse, that certification isn't necessary or important—choose another doctor.

• Ask questions that require evidence that the doctor knows the research on menopause. For example, "Would you tell me what the statistical risks are of endometrial cancer if I take X or Y brand of replacement estrogens?" or "Why exactly do you recommend X brand rather than Y brand of estrogens?" or "What exactly causes hot flashes, and why do I hear that replacement estrogens can get rid of them?" or "Should I take progestogen along with the estrogen? Why?"

These questions all require specific knowledge *and*—this is crucial—the ability to impart that knowledge to the patient in understandable language and in a way that will fully answer questions. In other words, you shouldn't walk out of the office with more questions than you had when you walked in.

If a doctor can't or won't answer specific questions, he or she is not doing the job that you are paying for.

• Decide whether the gynecologist is a person who wants patients to do what they're told (as one woman puts it, the "stick-with-me-kid" attitude) because it's easier for him or her to practice medicine that way, or is a person who expects the patient to make her own decisions based on the doctor's information and recommendations. One is, after all, paying good money for expert, educated advice. The physician is, theoretically at least, in the best position to know the benefits and harms of this, that, or the other treatment, and you may indeed want to follow the advice if you trust his or her judgment.

The only way to assess a doctor's attitude is to rely on your instincts; that is, if you feel patronized and mostly ignored by your gynecologist, you're probably right. The feeling has to originate somewhere, and you haven't fantasized an unpleasant experience. If you are legitimately angry when you walk out of the office, it would probably be smart not to walk back in.

Except in small towns, where there may be only one or two gynecologists, you can always find another doctor. The consumer of the service ought to be pleased with it—or take her business elsewhere.

The other way to decide about replacement estrogens is to read about the therapy in the responsible lay press. This means articles in established, high-quality publications that have a reputation for accuracy. For example, if an article on replacement estrogens appears in *Good Housekeeping* or *The New York Times,* you can assume that it was written by a responsible medical writer and checked by editors who make certain that all the facts are correct. The same type of story, however, in a pulp movie magazine probably is best left unread.

So too with book publishers. A company that has been in business for many years and prides itself on publishing quality books will not want to risk its reputation (and a possible lawsuit) printing medical information that is not factual and responsibly written.

Now to the heart of the matter about estrogen replacement therapy (ERT). First, it is important to note that there is still a good deal of controversy in the medical and research communities about the benefits and risks of ERT. It is generally safe and effective, but there are also hazards. Any medical therapy that is potent enough to cause a good effect is also potent enough to cause a bad effect, and the trick is to achieve a beneficial balance between the two.

As a woman approaches menopause, her ovaries produce less estradiol, one of the many types of estrogen, and ovulation and menstruation become sporadic. Meanwhile her adrenal glands begin to produce androstenedione, a weak androgen, which is converted to estrone, another type of estrogen. So a menopausal woman still has estrogen; it is just different from and not as potent as that produced by the ovaries.

The several different types of estrogen all have a similar chemical structure, and they all have a similar function: to cause estrus, the period of maximum sexual receptivity and fertility in mammals.

Progestogens are also variegated, but they are not as similar to each other as are estrogens. However, even as they differ, progestogens do have one function in common: They cause progestation, the preparation of the endometrium of the uterus for the fertilized ovum. In addition, they all have androgenic properties (those which mimic male hormones), which, as we shall see, *may* be a source of concern.

About menopause and estrogen production, "One thing is clearly true," says Dr. Bruce V. Stadel, a Medical Officer of the National Institute of Child Health and Human Development (NICHD), "is that the rate with which women lose calcium from their bones goes up. This can be stopped by giving estrogen."

A search of the medical literature reveals that calcium loss may not be stopped entirely, but it is undoubtedly true that the presence or absence of circulating estrogen makes a *significant* difference in the rate at which calcium is lost from the bones.

Says Stadel, "There is a critical point at which the skeletal system loses its structural integrity and starts to break easily. By giving estrogen, you can delay that point by 10, 15, or 20 years."

It is true that osteoporosis can be slowed somewhat by diet and exercise, but there is definite clinical proof that estrogen has a significant positive effect on bone and is a major benefit of ERT.

There are, however, important unanswered questions about ERT, says Stadel. The first is the issue of short-term versus long-term benefits. If estrogen could be tapered off after a year or so, when the short-term problems of menopause (such as hot flashes and diminished vaginal lubrication during sex) are no longer bothersome, what about the long-term problems such as osteoporosis?

Second, *who* should be treated with estrogens—all women, the ones with the most severe hot flashes and vaginitis, or only those who are at the highest risk of osteoporosis? And should only high-risk women receive ERT, or should they be the only ones on long-term therapy? And— just because thin, white women are at the highest risk for osteoporosis does *not* mean that other people are at no risk. So, should they or should they not start ERT, and if so, who and at what dose and for how long?

Stadel says that body weight can influence your decision. That is, the heavier you are, the more estrogen you are making on your own and the less you need replacement estrogens, but you are still not making as much as you were when you were menstruating. Therefore you are at *some* risk of osteoporosis and will have some amount of hot flashes and other menopausal symptoms.

Third, should ERT be given as treatment or for prevention? The theory behind treatment, says Stadel, is that when the problem for which someone is being treated has been resolved, the treatment is withdrawn. "Prophylaxis [prevention] implies that you go on forever because the risk of whatever you're trying to prevent will always exist."

Just as tooth decay is ever-present, and you can never stop brushing, the risk of osteoporosis is ever-present and even increases with age. Does this mean, then, that you must take estrogens forever?

"I don't know whether anyone could give a meaningful answer to that," says Stadel. "We don't have the data."

The only way to obtain sufficient data is to do very long-term studies (25 years or more) that compare the effect of menopause on women who have received replacement estrogens with those who have not. "The thought of doing such a study is daunting," says Stadel. "Although it's the only way to get definitive answers to very hard questions. But I doubt that right now the federal government or a private foundation would be willing to invest the $150 to $200 million that a study like that would cost."

What are the disadvantages of ERT? "For short-term therapy," says Stadel, "I don't know of any drawbacks."

For long-term therapy, the most prominent risk has been endometrial cancer. "Estrogen definitely increases the risk," says Stadel, "but this does not automatically preclude its use. It just means that the decision should be made especially carefully."

One should be careful, too, about reading the research data. The date the study was done is important because it will indicate the dose of estrogen used. Before the late 1970s the dose of estrogen tended to be much higher than it is now, higher, says Stadel, than what is needed to get most of the benefits of estrogen. And if the dose is higher than necessary, then the adverse effects will be more frequent and more severe than with the current low dose of estrogen.

So, if you're deciding in the mid-1980s to take ERT, you should discount reports of research published prior to 1980. "The excess risk reported in the past may be simply related to giving too much estrogen," says Stadel.

How great is the risk of endometrial cancer? "A several-fold increase," says Stadel. However, at a conference on ERT at the NICHD, Dr. Mortimer Lipsett, the institute's former director, reported the following statistics: The risk of endometrial cancer for *pre*menopausal women is 1 in 1000. The risk of endometrial cancer for *post*menopausal women who take estrogen *without* progestogen is 4 to 8 in 1000. The risk of endometrial cancer in *post*menopausal women who take estrogen *with* a seven- to ten-day course of progestogen is 1 in 1000. In other words, according to this report, progestogen lowers the risk to what it is in premenopausal women.

He went on to say that ERT is best given on a cyclical basis; that is, the estrogen should be periodically withdrawn and progestogen given in its place to induce menstrual bleeding and to mimic the natural menstrual cycle.

However—and this is a big however—there is no absolute proof that progestogen, given in conjunction with ERT, *significantly* alters the risk of endometrial cancer. Further, no one knows what the best estrogen/progestogen cycle is, nor is there a sufficient amount of data on the best dose of either hormone. That is:

• What is the minimum effective dose?
• At what dose does risk start to increase significantly?
• Is there a point beyond which the therapy should not continue, either because it is ineffective or unsafe, or both?

The risk of endometrial cancer, however small or unproven, creates a conflict: Is not a small risk of cancer better than a significant risk of osteoporosis? Isn't it better in the long run to have a hysterectomy, from which an otherwise healthy woman can recover completely, than to have a broken hip, from which many people never recover, or a perpetually shrunken spinal column?

Stadel responded to this dilemma by pointing out two important considerations about risk: "First, the woman who has characteristics indicative of osteoporosis is not likely to get into trouble from estrogen because she needs it. Giving too much estrogen or giving it to people who don't need it has been one of the primary problems.

"Second, almost all of the cases of endometrial cancer associated with estrogen appear to be a very low-grade form of cancer that does not metastasize [spread] rapidly and is usually curable by hysterectomy. If a woman is seeing a physician regularly and if she has any bleeding and if the physician is good and checks it out, the most she's likely to be faced with is the possibility of a hysterectomy."

Says Lipsett, "Endometrial cancer in postmenopausal women is 90 percent curable, mainly because women taking estrogen replacement therapy tend to be examined routinely and often. Doctors say they don't see 'galloping' uterine cancer in these women.''

Although, of course, everyone must decide alone which risks are acceptable and which are not, it seems logical to believe that a *small* risk of hysterectomy is far better than a *large* risk of crippling, permanent bone disease and fractures.

About breast cancer and ERT, Stadel says, "Many, many studies have been done about the relationship of breast cancer to replacement estrogens, and there is no proof that one has anything to do with the other."

Lipsett agrees. "Data on breast cancer in menopausal women taking estrogen replacement therapy is very inconclusive. There is no reason to believe, from a biological standpoint, that estrogen significantly increases the risk of breast cancer."

Stadel continued: "We do know enough about breast cancer, though, to know that it's theoretically reasonable to think that it *might* be affected by estrogens. So we're just going to have to continue to study the relationship. Because the disease is so common [it is the leading cause of cancer death among American women; seven percent of them will have it at some time during their lives], even a small increase in risk means that a significant number of women will be affected. So it's a problem we'll continue to study for a long time to come."

"But," and Stadel emphasized this: "if there *is* a relationship between breast cancer and ERT, it is definitely dose-related; that is, the more estrogen a woman takes, the higher her risk of cancer. My perception is that we could probably get an effective reduction of the osteoporosis risk with a dose that is low enough that, on the basis of the available evidence, the risk of breast cancer would not be materially increased."

In other words, a dose low enough to prevent the risk of breast cancer would also be sufficient to control osteoporosis. Stadel is careful to say that this is his professional opinion. There is as yet no clinical proof of the best dose of estrogen to balance the prevention of both osteoporosis and breast cancer. Again, long-term, very expensive studies are required to furnish such proof.

*   *   *

Since most of the increased risk of cancer in postmenopausal women seems to be connected to estrogen replacement, researchers have hypothesized that if some progestogen were given along with the estrogen, the risk could be reduced. Says Lipsett, "Anything that causes anovulatory periods [when no ovulation occurs] causes an increased risk of endometrial cancer because estrogen acts unopposed by progestogen. This is why it is important to give progestogen with the estrogen replacement therapy."

But it is also a fact that carcinogens (cancer-causing agents) act preferentially on growing tissue. Since the endometrium is renewed cyclically, the longer it undergoes this growth, the greater the risk of endometrial cancer. And since progestogen's main function is to stimulate the cells of the endometrium to multiply, it would seem that giving additional progestogen would increase rather than decrease the risk of endometrial cancer.

This is an apparent conflict, and in order to obtain tested proof that progestogen does indeed reduce the risk of cancer when given in conjunction with ERT, long-term studies comparing the two types of hormone therapy will need to be done. But in so doing, serious ethical dilemmas would be created. Among them:

• If estrogen alone is strongly linked to increased risk of cancer, would it be permissible to ask some people to undergo that treatment?

• Who should be recruited as research subjects, and how should they be compensated if they develop cancer or another serious illness as a result of the treatment?

• If animal studies show clearly that one or the other hormone therapy is safer and/or more beneficial, why should research subjects be given the other therapy?

• Yet, human studies *have* to be done because human and animal physiology, although similar in some aspects, is not the same, and because a treatment that works on animals does not automatically mean that it will work on humans.

"In theory," says Stadel, "if you give progestogen, you get better shedding of the endometrium at menstruation, and you're less likely to get cancer because the endometrial tissue just isn't there. Whether this works or not to prevent cancer has not been determined. One thinks it should, but no one has actually done a study to prove that progestogen prevents endometrial cancer."

Investigators are just now beginning to look at the effect of progestogen when combined with estrogen as replacement therapy. Progestogen inhibits or curbs the unopposed action of estrogen. Thus, if estrogen is indeed in some way responsible for the development of endometrial cancer, then the addition of progestogen to the estrogen therapy should theoretically lower the risk of cancer.

Most medical references say that progestogen should be given for seven to ten days each month in the lowest effective dose. It may also be effective for the treatment of endometrial hyperplasia (an abnormal increase in the number of *normal* cells). This is a noncancerous condition, but it is frightening because it causes bleeding, and one reference says that treatment with progestogen can be effective in 95 percent of the cases, thus obviating the need for surgery.

Progestogen may also enhance the bone-sparing effects of ERT by increasing bone mineral content.

Like all treatments, progestogen has its dark side. It may impair glucose tolerance, causing diabetes-like symptoms, although this doesn't seem to be a significant problem. There seems to be a good deal of controversy about whether progestogen increases or decreases the risk of breast cancer, and as there is no proof one way or the other, there is little point in speculation. Certainly there are no definite indications that it does.

"So what's the bottom line in all this controversy?" asks Stadel. He answers his own question: "There's no doubt that hormone replacement therapy, either estrogen alone or estrogen with progestogen, is a safe and effective way to reduce the incidence of osteoporosis; that is, it slows the process. The question then becomes, 'Who should be treated?' Those are questions to which there are no simple answers. My view is that when the dose is low enough to control symptoms only and if the woman is getting regular examinations, the risk of serious illness or death is quite small, particularly in view of the benefits."

A low daily dose usually means 0.625 mg to 1.25 mg of the type of estrogen contained in Premarin, the most frequently prescribed brand of conjugated estrogens. The best way to prescribe ERT, says Stadel, is to start with the lowest possible dose and then increase it in very small increments until the symptoms stop.

However, you must be carefully monitored, and should not be left on estrogen indefinitely for menopausal symptoms. The dose should then be gradually tapered off to where symptoms are still controlled and the osteoporotic process prevented as much as possible. This is not a simple task, mostly because there are so few medical guidelines. Thus, it is extremely important that you choose a gynecologist who not only keeps up with the research on ERT but who is interested in the issue and is willing to devote the time necessary to monitor you.

Most of the research that has been published about ERT since 1980 concentrates on correlating the therapy with the risk of various types of cancer, but there have been other studies as well—literally hundreds of them about ERT, with or without progestogen. A computer search of this medical literature reveals that ERT does what it is designed to do; that is, it relieves the unpleasant symptoms of menopause, and it prevents some degree of bone loss. These facts are now well established, and no one in the research community disagrees about them. However, there is still much controversy about ERT and thus many questions worth investigating. Following is a sample of current research:

• At a conference in England in September 1983 on the calcification of bone tissue, C. Christiansen reported the results of a study comparing women with serious osteoporosis to those with a mild case of the disease, and their response to estrogen therapy.

He studied 88 postmenopausal women for two years and measured the calcium content of their bones every three months. The rate of bone loss was dose-dependent; that is, the rates at which calcium was depleted from bones depended not on whether the women were rapid or nonrapid bone losers before the ERT but on the amount of estrogen they received.

Although this study provides no specific guidelines on precisely how much estrogen to prescribe, it does indicate that physicians should not only be particularly alert to dose levels, they must also keep track of the osteoporotic process.

• Kreiger, Kelsey, et al., studied the relationship of hip fractures to past exposure to estrogen. They compared women who were admitted to hospital with hip fractures with women in the same hospital who were admitted for other reasons. The cases (women with fractures) and controls (other women) were closely matched for age, menopausal status, and other variables.

"Fewer cases of hip fracture than controls had been exposed [to estrogen], exposure time was shorter than for controls, the cases had breast fed their children for shorter duration, and they more often had had both ovaries removed. Also, the cases were found to weigh less than the controls."[1]

The authors concluded that ERT can prevent hip fractures, as can intact ovaries and excess weight.

• In an important study Hulka, Chambless, et al., looked at the relationship of ERT to breast cancer. They compared 199 postmenopausal breast cancer patients with 451 patients who were hospitalized for another reason and 852 healthy people for past use of estrogen.

"Estrogen did not increase the breast cancer risk for women with a surgical menopause [oophorectomy]. Among women with a natural menopause, estrogens administered by all routes were associated with a breast cancer risk of 1.7 and 1.8.* There was no coherent pattern of changing risks with varying durations of use, different daily dosages, years since first use of estrogen, or years since most recent use. When women who usually received estrogen by injection were excluded, the risk estimates for oral estrogens were 1.3 (case subjects compared to healthy nonhospitalized women) and 1.2 (case subjects compared to hospital control subjects). These increases were not statistically significant."[2]

Since a risk factor of 1.2 or 1.3 is so insignificant as to be almost nonexistent, and since almost no one receives ERT by injection, we can conclude from this study that estrogen does not increase the risk of breast cancer.

---

*A risk factor of 1 means there is no increased risk. A risk factor of 2 means that twice as much risk exists.

• P. D. Saville noted that the administration of various forms of estrogen to postmenopausal women definitely prevents some deterioration of the skeleton. This fact was not news, but the investigator went on to say that, "The safety of long-term estrogen administration has not been established by large-scale controlled studies. Therefore, hormone treatment should be reserved for patients with symptoms of estrogen deficiency or for subsets of persons at increased risk of osteoporotic bone fractures. These include fair-skinned or lightweight persons, smokers, heavy drinkers, persons on prolonged corticosteroid therapy, those with early menopause [before age 40], and those with rheumatoid arthritis."[3]

In other words, ERT is beneficial for some women, but the therapy is not appropriate for all, and no one yet knows what the ultimate effects of long-term therapy (more than five years) will be.

• In another study about estrogen and osteoporosis, Horsman, Jones, et al., found that, "In postmenopausal women, the reduction in the rate of cortical bone loss in response to estrogen therapy depends on the dose administered."[4]

• Sherman, Wallace, and Bean investigated the relationship of obesity and ERT. The report appears in the April 15, 1983 issue of *Cancer*.

The researchers found that there is a positive correlation between breast cancer and obesity: Fat women are more likely to get breast cancer than thin ones. And since postmenopausal obese women tend to manufacture more of their own estrogen than thin women, the investigators thought there might be a similar correlation between exogenous estrogen* and breast cancer.

They compared 113 postmenopausal breast cancer patients to similar women who did not have breast cancer and found that neither taking estrogen at menopause nor body weight were significantly associated with breast cancer risk. However, *among estrogen users,* the risk of breast cancer was significantly higher for overweight women. However, among

---

*Endogenous estrogen is that produced by the woman herself; exogenous estrogen is that supplied from outside the body, as in ERT.

the women who got breast cancer, the thinner ones developed it an average of seven years earlier than heavier women.

This study suggests very strongly that obese women should think carefully before embarking on a course of ERT because if they do take estrogens, they are more likely to get breast cancer than thin women, but they will most likely get it at a later age. Luckily, obese women are the least likely to suffer from the unpleasant effects of menopause and thus are least likely to take replacement estrogens.

The clinical practice aspects of ERT are somewhat different from the research aspects. That is, the practicing physician must make judgments based not only on what he or she knows to be scientifically true or statistically relevant but also on the general health and other characteristics of the patient. The doctor needs to take into account the risks and benefits for that particular patient at that particular time in her life.

The physician is, however, not without guidelines for recommending one or another course of action. For instance, a woman who is hypertensive (has high blood pressure) should be especially carefully watched because ERT *may* increase her blood pressure. This is also true of a woman who is a likely candidate for gallbladder disease.

There still seems to be an unresolved relationship between ERT and hypertension. Theoretically, estrogen should make blood pressure go up because of its effect on certain other body chemicals, and sometimes it does, but when the estrogen is withdrawn, blood pressure immediately drops to normal.

Lipsett says, "Postmenopausal women on estrogen replacement therapy have not shown an elevated blood pressure, but further research is needed because premenopausal women who take oral contraceptives have a two to five percent increase in blood pressure. This hypertension is transient [temporary], however, and blood pressure goes back to normal when the woman stops taking the birth control pills."

The risk of gallstones increases somewhat (2.5 percent) with ERT, especially if the woman is obese, when the risk is even higher.

Studies have shown, however, that there is *no* increased risk of psychiatric disorders, myocardial infarction (heart attack), cerebrovascular accidents (stroke), pulmonary embolism (blood clot in the lung), or diabetes.

Clare Erdman, writing in a medical text on menopause, says that the physician should carefully evaluate all patients who are to have ERT. This evaluation should include a complete medical and gynecologic history, a physical and pelvic examination, and an endometrial biopsy, which she says is *mandatory*.

An endometrial biopsy consists of removing a small amount of endometrial tissue by passing a small tube through the vagina into the uterine cavity. Low suction is applied when the tube touches the endometrial wall. The procedure takes about five or ten minutes, and although it isn't terribly painful, it isn't much fun, either. When the suction is applied, you may feel as though you are having severe menstrual cramps. When the suction is turned off, the cramps stop, and you *may* have a dull abdominal ache and slight vaginal bleeding for the rest of the day. Some women have no aftereffects at all.

The tissue is then examined under the microscope, and the pathologist looks for abnormal or precancerous cells. If they are present, you should *not* start on replacement estrogen.

Erdman says that, in addition to an abnormal endometrial biopsy, there are several conditions under which a menopausal woman should *absolutely not* take estrogen. They are:

- Undiagnosed vaginal bleeding
- Acute liver disease
- Chronic impaired liver function
- Vascular thrombosis (blood clots)
- Neuro-ophthalmologic vascular disease (abnormality of the blood vessels in the eye)
- Existing breast cancer
- Chronic thrombophlebitis

She also lists some relative contraindications, those conditions that must be evaluated for severity before prescribing ERT. They are: preexisting and chronic hypertension, fibrocystic disease of the breasts, benign tumors of the uterus (such as fibroids), severe varicose veins, gallbladder disease, severe obesity, and smoking.

The physician should also consider the woman's age. In general, all women who have premature menopause, if they are not obese, should take estrogen from the time of menopause (whether it occurs naturally or as a result of the surgical removal of the ovaries) until they are 50 years old. Obese women do not need ERT (or only very low doses if they are only moderately fat) because they produce their own supply of the hormone.

Not all postmenopausal women need ERT, and not all need the same amount. Again, in general, thin, small-framed white women who smoke and who weigh less than 120 pounds should be on long-term ERT because they are at the greatest risk of osteoporosis. Other menopausal women should take ERT only if they need it, that is, only if they are having problems with menopause and then only on a short-term basis—for no longer than five years. At the end of that time they should be evaluated for osteoporotic changes.

ERT is generally given by mouth. Injectable estrogens are available for women who, for one reason or another, can't take the hormone orally, but the dose is higher, the action is more prolonged, and it costs more.

Once a woman starts to take replacement estrogens, she should go to the doctor every six to 12 months for a check of her breasts, blood pressure, and pelvic and reproductive organs. After the initial endometrial biopsy, it is not necessary to repeat the test *unless* the woman has had vaginal bleeding. Then it is *imperative* that the cells be examined again.

One-third of all postmenopausal women on ERT will have uterine bleeding which is dose- and use-related. That is, the higher the dose of estrogen and the longer the woman continues the therapy, the greater the likelihood of bleeding. Most often the bleeding is transient and utterly benign, but it still requires an endometrial biopsy. Sometimes bleeding can be controlled by combining the estrogen therapy with progestogen.

If the physician says to a woman on ERT with vaginal bleeding that a biopsy isn't necessary, or if he or she says, "We'll watch it for a while and see what happens," she should walk out of the office and find herself another doctor.

Endometrial cancer is highly curable if treated in the early stages, and the only way to diagnose it is by biopsy. A woman is doing herself a great disservice if she doesn't get to the doctor and insist on a biopsy *as soon as* she sees bleeding. THIS IS CRUCIALLY IMPORTANT.

As we have already noted, estrogen's effect on bone is dose-related, and with regard to this Erdman notes: "Low-dose estrogen therapy does arrest and retard bone resorption up to 8 years if therapy is begun shortly after the loss of ovarian estrogen; however, more longevity studies are needed before these observations may be used as the premise for long-term therapy. Such therapy does prevent the development of bone fragility and reduces the incidence of fractures. Discontinuation of the early initiated estrogen therapy often results in a rapid loss of bone density similar to that observed in nonuser individuals."[5]

This appears to mean that ERT, if discontinued too soon, is as good as useless, that is, that the treatment, once started for the control of osteoporosis, should be maintained to prevent rapid bone loss. But maintained for how long and for which women? These questions still stump practicing physicians because medical research has provided no definitive answers.

Erdman comments on the dilemma: "Despite the effect of long-term estrogen therapy on bone, there is still the question of whether all postmenopausal women need estrogen therapy, especially now that progestins* have been found to enhance new bone formation in postmenopausal women. Most clinicians do not place all postmenopausal women on replacement therapy to protect 25–30% of the population. They would recommend that Caucasian [white] women with small body frames who smoke or were castrated prior to age 40 be started on prophylactic [preventive] replacement therapy."[6]

Since estrogen is the major active ingredient in oral contraceptives, and since cardiovascular problems have been the

---

*Progestins are the same as progestogens. It's a shortened form of the same word.

most significant and serious adverse effect of these pills, it would be logical to look at the relationship between ERT and the incidence of cardiovascular disease in postmenopausal women. In fact, there is a negative correlation; that is, ERT seems to prevent cardiovascular disease, at least to some extent. Says Erdman, "Synthetic estrogens in oral contraceptives are associated with a high incidence of deep vein thrombosis and myocardial infarction after age 40. Despite these well-documented observations in premenopausal women, long-term estrogen therapy in postmenopausal women has not been associated with an increased incidence of occlusive arterial or venous thromboembolic disease [blood clots in the arteries or veins]. This is somewhat surprising since risk factors such as hypertension, hyperlipidemia [an excess of fatty substances circulating in the bloodstream], and obesity are common in menopausal women. Many investigators attribute these observations to the predominant use of *natural estrogens* during estrogen replacement therapy."[7]

Each woman must evaluate the pros and cons of ERT for herself. You should do as much reading as you can, ask the advice of a doctor you know and can trust because he or she is a competent practitioner, and then you must make the decision—which is not irrevocable. ERT can be stopped as well as started. All you have to do is throw away the pills. They're your pills, and it's your body.

Chapter Four

FRACTURES

*O*steoporotic bones break easily, and fracture is the most serious consequence of the disease. Breaking a bone is an ever-present danger and can mean months of pain and disability, even permanent crippling. And for 20 percent of those who fracture their hips, it means death within a year.

The risk of fracture is directly proportional to bone density; that is, the stronger and more compact the bone, the less likely it is to break. Fractures tend to occur where there is a large proportion of trabecular or spongy bone and in places where the bone itself is most vulnerable, for example, the neck of the femur or radius. People who have already had one osteoporotic fracture, even a microscopic one, have a higher than average risk of future fractures.

In women, as a rule, the first fracture after menopause is the wrist (Colles fracture), then one or more vertebrae. Since the risk of fracture increases as soon as bone mass starts to decrease, a menopausal woman who has done nothing to prevent osteoporosis can expect to break something soon after her periods stop if she is not careful. In men, there is no increase in the incidence of Colles fracture, and there are no statistics available for the incidence of spontaneous compression fracture of the vertebrae due to osteoporosis. This is not to say that men don't break their backs; they do, but it's difficult to distinguish between spontaneous fractures and those arising from physical exertion or accidents. The incidence of hip fracture in men increases with age, but the rate of increase is slower than that of women. By the time a woman is 80 years old, there is a 25 percent chance that she will have had at least one fracture.

The treatment for osteoporotic fractures is the same as it is for any other fracture, but the success rate is markedly poorer; that is, the fracture does not heal as completely as it does in younger people because old tissue of any kind does not heal as rapidly as young tissue, and if there is diminished absorption of calcium, healing will be further delayed.

When a bone breaks, there is major damage to the bone as well as to surrounding tissues, and the whole area immediately swells and hurts terribly. The bone is severed, of course, but marrow, the substance in the hollow of long bones in which both red and white blood cells are manufactured, leaks out as well. Blood vessels are also severed, and if the fracture is particularly severe, the surrounding muscle might also be torn.

The healing process, however, begins immediately as long as there is no uncontrollable hemorrhage (which is very rare in osteoporotic fractures). The first stage of healing, which begins right after the fracture and lasts until cartilage formation starts, is called the stage of inflammation. This is the time when there is the most acute pain and swelling and when the fracture must be reduced. Reduction means fitting the two ends of the bone back together and immobilizing them.

Closed reduction means that the two bone fragments are manipulated through the skin and then immobilized by casting, pinning, or traction. Casting is the application of a plaster cast with which almost everyone is familiar. Pinning is the insertion of a stainless steel pin or nail through the two bone fragments to hold them together more satisfactorily than a cast alone. Pins are sometimes used when a cast is not practical (for example, in a hip fracture) and sometimes in conjunction with a cast. Traction is weight applied to one end of the broken bone to keep it aligned during the first part of the healing process, usually on a bone that has to bear weight, such as a leg, hip, or back.

Open reduction means that the orthopedist makes an incision and manipulates the bone fragments from inside. He or she then immobilizes the bone as described.

During the stage of inflammation, which lasts for three or four days, a blood clot (hematoma) forms at the fracture site, and some of the bone at the two jagged edges dies because it has lost the continuity of blood supply. There is also intense activity on the part of almost all the unicellular structures of the body; all of one's defense mechanisms spring into action. Certain white cells remove dead tissue, cell by cell; fibroblasts (cells that help form connective tissue) weave an intricate grid to form the blood clot; osteoclasts also remove dead cells; osteoblasts start forming new cartilage and bone cells; and other cells work to constrict blood vessels in the bone marrow and elsewhere to prevent uncontrolled bleeding.

The second stage, called the soft callus stage, is also active. Calluses, composed mostly of cartilage, form both in and around the bone. The external callus, formed by the active proliferation of osteoblasts on the periosteum (the tough outer sheath covering the bone), creates a kind of protective bridge that helps immobilize the two ends of the shattered bone. The internal soft callus also holds the bone fragments together, and it serves as a pathway for the reestablishment of blood circulation.

This period of cartilage formation lasts about three or four weeks and is followed by the stage of hard callus in which the callus gradually converts to bone. All this time the osteoclasts remove dead bone while osteoblasts create new bone. The hard callus stage lasts from about three or four weeks after the break until three or four months later in the average adult. In a person with osteoporosis the process can take twice as long.

In addition to carrying off dead bone cells, the osteoclasts remodel the new bone. The bump formed by the external callus has turned into bone, but that is slowly smoothed away by osteoclasts. When the two edges of the broken bone are completely fused by the formation of new bone, healing is complete.

Doctors no longer consider a broken back as medically serious as they used to, although it is by no means a trivial matter, and to the patient it is frightening and incapacitating.

This change in attitude has several bases. First, less than

five percent of all broken vertebrae also result in damage to the spinal cord. The spinal cord and the spine are not the same thing. The spine is a column of vertebral bones running down the center of the back, interspersed with discs (figure 3). The spinal cord is a bundle of nerve tissues arising in the brain and running through the center of the spinal column.

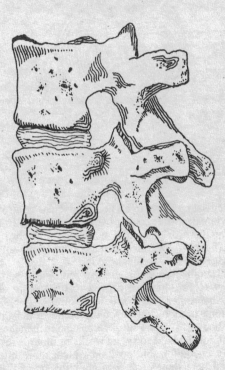

FIGURE #3
Three Vertebrae Showing Discs

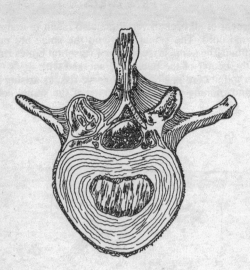

FIGURE #4
Cross Section of Vertebrae

This nerve tissue is vital to all neuromuscular control, and if severed will cause irreversible paralysis. Damage to the spinal column may or may not mean that the cord is also damaged (figure 4). We shall discuss how to prevent spinal cord damage and how to diagnose it.

Second, laminectomy, the surgical removal of part of one or more vertebrae, has not proved to be a more effective treatment than other, less drastic, measures.

Third, long immobilization of the spine in a tight-fitting jacket or body cast is no longer considered beneficial, and the patient doesn't have to spend weeks or months restrained in a highly uncomfortable position which, more often than not, caused persistent back pain after the original fracture had healed.

Most fractures occur in the mid to lower back, not only because of the peculiarities of the anatomy of the spine but also because this is the area of greatest stress. Doctors still argue about the advantages of conservative (nonsurgical) versus surgical treatment of spinal fractures.

Says R. Bruce Heppenstall, "Several spinal centers in the United States have been taking a more aggressive approach [than those that advocate intermittent bed rest as described in Chapter 2] and advocating operative stabilization of the fractures and early mobilization of the patients in an attempt to prevent secondary complications. This approach is similar to the early-weight-bearing concept in the treatment of fractures that has emerged during the past two decades. There is no doubt that the theory of early mobilization in association with operative stabilization has significantly changed the outlook of many patients with spinal fractures."[1]

In other words, getting people up and about as soon as possible is not only medically advantageous, the patient likes it better. And no wonder! If one were given a choice between an operation and the promise of a relatively short time of being totally immobilized in bed, or no operation and months of a regimen that required hours each day of lying flat in bed, most people would choose the former.

Just as getting up as soon as possible after surgery has definite psychologic benefits, so it has physiologic ones as well. The longer one stays in bed, the greater one's chances of a wide variety of complications, such as: blood clots in the leg that can break off and travel to the heart, lungs, and brain—with possibly fatal results; muscle weakness that progresses to atrophy (shrinkage); hypostatic pneumonia, which results from incomplete exchange of oxygen and carbon dioxide in the lungs or the incomplete exhalation of anesthesia; and the further loss of bone tissue that always accompanies prolonged immobilization. The last is particularly serious for people with osteoporosis, who absolutely cannot afford to lose more bone tissue.

People on prolonged bed rest are also prone to bed sores that are likely to become infected. They may have to be catheterized,* either continuously or intermittently and often get urinary tract infections. And it's not uncommon for them to become depressed to the point of despondence.

---

*Urinary catheterization is the passage of a sterile tube through the urethra into the bladder to release urine.

The spinal column is a series of vertebrae, each one with a hollow center through which runs the spinal cord, stacked one atop the other, interspersed with intervertebral discs. These discs are composed of fibrocartilage material which increases in size and thickness as the size and thickness of the vertebrae increase from top to bottom. The discs lengthen the spinal column and function as shock absorbers between the vertebrae, much as shock absorbers on a car cushion the passengers from the jolts delivered by ruts and potholes. The cartilaginous material also has the capacity to absorb large quantities of water, a quality that enhances their shock-absorbing ability. As a person grows older, the discs lose their capacity to hold water, and it is this, as well as the increasing porousness of the trabecular or spongy bone of the vertebrae, that increases the incidence of compression fractures. Further, as the discs decrease in size as the person ages, the spinal column itself shortens (figure 5).

The spinal column is highly flexible; one has only to watch ballet dancers or gymnasts in action to realize the full ca-

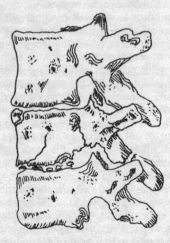

FIGURE #5
Compression Fracture of Vertebrae

pability of this structural support system. The vertebrae themselves (that is, each separate bone) cannot be flexed, but the discs, muscles, and ligaments that intersperse and surround the spinal column are highly flexible. The column is not uniformly supple along its entire length. The upper and lower parts (those in the neck and lower back) bend more easily than do those in the middle where the ribs are attached. The column is also capable of rotation, again more easily in the upper and lower parts than in the middle. However, one can get the spinal column to do only so much, and eventually it will break. The older one gets, the weaker the bones, the more rigid the discs, the more likely is fracture.

Spinal fractures are characterized as either stable or unstable. Stability means that the fracture or dislocation will not become displaced during repair; that is, the fragments will remain aligned. Instability means that it is possible that during treatment the bone fragments will shift, thus making healing more difficult and possibly even causing damage to the spinal cord.

In treating a broken back, the physician must know exactly what happened, that is, *how* the injury occurred. Diagnosing the fracture depends to a great extent on knowing the type and force of motion that caused the injury. Bending over to pick up something off the floor will produce a very different kind of injury than will being thrown sideways in the back seat of a car during a collision. The doctor also needs to know what the person felt immediately after the injury (pain, numbness, tingling, "pins and needles," etc.) to determine if there is also spinal cord injury. Treatment of a broken back with spinal cord injury is very different from a relatively uncomplicated fracture.

What happens immediately after the injury can be crucial to the success of the treatment. And the most crucial part of the immediate post-injury scenario is the way the person is moved. The entire back must be supported on a flat surface during transport to the emergency room. Rescue squad members and many policemen know exactly how to move someone with a back injury; most "ordinary" people do not.

All serious back injuries should be attended to at once. Usually the pain will be severe enough to make one grateful for a hospital, but once in a while the pain starts as only a mild, dull ache that gradually increases in intensity. Those who refuse to go to the doctor in the presence of not-very-severe pain are making a mistake. The earlier treatment is begun (that is, the sooner the spinal column is immobilized), the better the healing process will be.

The person must have a neurologic as well as an orthopedic examination as soon as possible, because only with specific tests and examinations can the extent of nervous system damage be assessed. If the emergency room physician does not do a neurologic examination or send for a qualified neurologist, the injured person should insist that this be done. He or she should also insist on being seen by an orthopedic specialist, not just the general resident on duty in the emergency room. It's not always easy, when one is in pain, scared, and intimidated by the hustle-bustle of the emergency room, to know if the care provided is competent, or even adequate. Some things that you can do to protect yourself are:

• Ask the examining doctor if he or she is a board certified orthopedist (or neurologist). If the answer is no, request a specialist; the chief of the department is a good place to start.

• Pay attention to what's being done to you or asked of you.* A neurologic examination consists of asking very specific questions about the nature of the injury, and the sensations immediately following, as well as a good amount of poking and prodding to test reflexes and responses to various stimuli. *Ask* if what the doctor is doing is a neurologic examination.

• Insist on X-rays. If the emergency room physician says, "It's nothing but a strain or pulled muscle," insist on X-rays anyway. Although not all vertebral fractures are apparent on X-ray, a break surely won't be diagnosed if pictures aren't taken.

The X-ray process is so important that Heppenstall says, "Patients with thoracolumbar spinal injuries [mid to lower

---

*If you are unconscious, or conscious but not thinking clearly, and alone, you have no choice but to trust the care provided. If you are with a patient who is unconscious, act as the advocate for that person and insist on all the actions listed above.

back] frequently are brought into the emergency room during the early hours of the morning, and it is imperative that the physician accompany the patient to the radiology department in order to supervise the roentgenographic* evaluation. It is best to leave the patient on the stretcher rather than to transfer him to the regular roentgenographic table. The first view that should be obtained is a straight lateral [from the side] roentgenographic view of the thoracolumbar spine. This will provide insight into the presence of an unstable spinal fracture. If no evidence of spinal fracture or dislocation is revealed, the technician can then proceed to a thorough evaluation of the entire thoracolumbar spine. The anteroposterior [front to back] view must be obtained with the patient in the supine [lying flat on the back] position. If a physician does not supervise the roentgenographic evaluation, a patient may inadvertently be placed in the seated position to obtain various roentgenographic views, which is contraindicated with this type of fracture."[2]

In other words, the physician must make certain that not only are the X-rays taken correctly but that the patient is not permitted to sit up. If Heppenstall, writing in a major medical text on fractures, specifically reminds physicians not to leave X-ray technicians alone with patients with possibly broken backs, two things must be true: (1) it must be exceedingly important to lie flat at all times; and (2) he must have had a good deal of experience with patients being asked to sit up. Contrary to popular belief, one *can* sit up with a broken back, but it's obviously extremely unwise to do so.

The choice of treatment of vertebral fracture depends on whether it is stable or unstable. Flexion fracture, very common in people with osteoporosis, is a type of stable injury that arises from overflexion of the spine caused, for example, by bending over to pick up something too heavy. In a person with severe osteoporosis, "too heavy" might be nothing more than a dropped fork. It is the act of bending over suddenly one time too many that causes the fracture, not the weight of the retrieved object.

---

*Wilhelm Roentgen discovered the X-ray in 1895, for which he won the first Nobel Prize in physics. *Roentgenograph* is the medical term for X-ray.

There is sudden pain in one definite spot, and the urge to "splint" the fracture by not moving is almost overwhelming. Besides, it hurts too much to move.

In most cases the treatment is nothing more than the extended periods of intermittent rest and activity already described, although sometimes the person is in mild extension traction for the first two or three weeks. This consists of lying on the back encased in a system of weights and pulleys so that the spine is fixed in a mildly stretched-out (extended) position.

Extension fracture is another example of a stable injury, although it isn't as common as flexion fracture. In this case, the vertebra breaks when the spine is suddenly extended. The injury usually occurs in the mid to lower back, and depending on the extent of the fracture, the person can be treated conservatively (no cast) or with a body cast for the first few weeks until the fracture begins to heal. Then activity can be gradually increased, but a fairly supportive back brace should be worn.

Axial load (burst) fracture means that not only has the vertebra broken, it has comminuted (separated) into two or more pieces. These unstable breaks require more serious treatment because there may be spinal cord injury as well as damage to the bone. The first line of treatment is to take the pressure off the spinal cord and then to immobilize the spine until the pieces of the vertebra fuse. This often involves surgery, perhaps fusing the broken vertebra to the ones above and below it in order to strengthen the entire area. However, spinal fusion is not as common as it used to be because new surgical techniques have taken its place. In any event, the person with an axial load fracture will almost certainly be in a body cast for several weeks, and he or she may even have temporary paralysis below the level of the fracture if the vertebral fragments damaged the spinal cord. After the parts of the vertebra have fused, the remainder of the treatment is much the same as it is for any other type of broken back.

It is almost as natural as breathing to throw your arms out horizontally to regain balance to forestall a fall. It's a reflex action that often works because the force of throwing out the arms counteracts the force of gravity. You stumble or trip, your heart lurches, and that's all there is to it.

However, when the force of gravity is stronger than the counterbalancing arm pinwheeling, a fall is inevitable, and if you land on your outstretched hand in just the right way, your wrist breaks.

The radius is the inner and shorter of the two bones leading from the elbow to the hand (figure 6). It partially rotates around the other bone, the ulna, and thus is more likely to break at the wrist end. This is called a Colles fracture (figure 7)—first described by the Irish surgeon Abraham Colles in

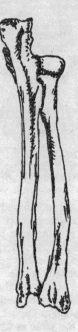

FIGURE #6
Radius and Ulna

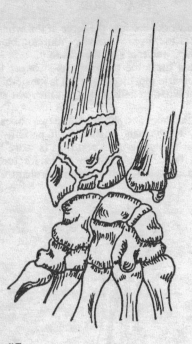

FIGURE #7
Comminuted Colles Fracture (Radius) Wrist

1814—and is one of the most common fractures in all people, but especially those with osteoporosis. When the head of the radius also breaks into two or more pieces, the result is a comminuted (separated and fragmented) Colles fracture. The extent of the injury depends on the position of the wrist at impact; the physical strength of the bones themselves, as well as the muscles and ligaments that support them; the magnitude of the force at impact; and the rate of speed at which the stress was applied at impact.

The principle is much the same as what happens during an automobile accident. The faster the car is going, the worse the impact will be. The greater the strength of the car, the less the damage. The more stationary the person in the car is (that is, the better the seat belt), the less he or she will be tossed about on impact, and the less severe the injury.

The older the person, the more likely he or she is to break a wrist when falling, and the more severe the injury is likely to be. Further, once an elderly person with osteoporosis breaks a wrist, he or she will be more likely to break the same wrist again after an injury of even less force. In other words, the site of the fracture, even after it has healed as well as it ever will, is always less strong than the never-fractured bone. In fact, the likelihood of a second fracture increases threefold.

According to Heppenstall, the rate of wrist fracture in postmenopausal women is 54 per 10,000—four times the rate for hip fractures and about five times the rate for the general population. Although types of wrist fractures vary tremendously depending on the factors already listed, they generally fall into three categories:

• a simple fracture of the radius itself not involving the surface of the joint;*
• a fracture involving the joint surface but without displacement of the bone fragments; and
• a comminuted fracture when the bone fragments are displaced and the line of the fracture runs into the joint.

Heppenstall describes the prognosis for complete healing of a Colles fracture: "In general, the greater the degree of articular [joint] surface involvement, the greater the initial displacement, the more comminuted the fracture site, the more involved the ulnar side of the wrist, the worse the prognosis."[3]

In other words, the "messier" the fracture site, the harder it will be to heal completely. In addition, the greater the degree of joint involvement and the more imperfect the even-

---

*This can be confusing because people think of the wrist itself as a joint. However, the radius ends at the joint with the metacarpals, and a clean break of the bone itself does not involve the joint, even though it appears to from the outside because people think of the whole "bracelet" area as the wrist.

tual healing, the more likely the person is to suffer from arthritis in that wrist as time goes by.

A Colles fracture is sometimes called a "dinner fork" fracture because of the pattern of bone displacement and swelling. The wrist appears "humped up," much like the upward bend in a fork at the joining between the tines and the shaft of the handle. A Colles fracture hurts immediately and severely, and there is considerable swelling. X-rays must be taken, of course, but even to an unpracticed eye, one look at the swollen and misshapen wrist will "diagnose" a Colles fracture—it's that distinctive in appearance. Also many people say that they feel the bone "give way" on impact and realize immediately that they have broken their wrist.

Treatment of a Colles fracture differs depending on the nature and extent of the injury, but all fractures must be reduced and immobilized.

In closed reduction, the physician manipulates the bones through the skin, X-rays the radius, ulna, and joint to see that the alignment is correct, applies a cast, and then lets nature take its course. Naturally the person is anesthetized throughout all this because the process of reduction hurts mightily. The type of anesthesia used depends on the extent of the injury and on age and general health. Three types of anesthesia are generally used:

• local, in which only the wrist itself is "numbed" with Xylocaine or another similar drug;
• extremity block, in which the entire arm is numbed; and
• general, in which the person is rendered unconscious.

If open reduction and/or pinning is required, general anesthesia is the only choice.

When the fracture has been reduced, and the X-ray shows that all the fragments are back in proper alignment, the entire area must be immobilized until the fracture heals. There are a number of ways of doing this, the most common of which is a plaster cast. Heppenstall says that the type of cast used (long or short, heavy or light) is less important than adhering to general casting principles, of which he lists three:

• No cast should extend beyond the knuckles in order that the person have full range of motion of his or her fingers.

• Any, even minor, swelling or neurologic symptoms (numbness, tingling, paralysis, etc.) requires immediate splitting of the cast.

• The fracture should be X-rayed at periodic intervals; for example, three days, ten days, and three weeks after the injury, to see that the bone fragments remain in alignment.

The reader might wonder why medical principles of casting are included in a book for the layperson. "Why," one could ask, "should I worry about what the doctor should be doing when I have to concentrate on getting someone to drive me around and even get help to button my buttons?"

The answer is that knowing what *should* be done provides a cushion of safety and can prevent future serious medical problems. The three principles are all designed to prevent damage and deformity to the wrist, fingers, and elbow and thus are of deep concern to the person dragging around a heavy plaster cast. For example, if one doesn't have free and complete use of the fingers, the knuckles will "freeze," the muscles will atrophy, and there will be permanent loss of range of motion. The person with a broken wrist *must* flex his or her fingers frequently enough to keep the joints fluid and fully functional. This hurts. In the beginning, it hurts like hell, and the temptation not to move the fingers is strong. But it takes only a short time, sometimes as little as a week, for joints to start to stiffen, and the more time that goes by, the more permanent the damage. Although most orthopedists will not put on a cast that covers the fingers, not all physicians are perfectly competent, and if the person with a broken wrist wakes up to find his or her fingers covered in plaster, he or she should question the rationale and request that the cast be shortened. Moreover, some doctors simply don't think to tell their patients how important it is to constantly exercise the fingers. They send them home from the hospital with a pat on the back, in the belief that the patient will know what to do.

With regard to the second principle, swelling within the

cast is dangerous because it can cut off circulation, and if severe and long-lasting enough, can cause gangrene. If tissue swells inside a cast, it has only a finite amount of room in which to expand; when it uses up all the available space, the force and direction of the expansion reverse because soft tissue is more yielding than the hard plaster cast. Thus, small blood vessels and cells become compressed and blood flow is cut off. Tissue that doesn't have access to blood flow dies, and gangrene is simply the word for death and putrefaction of tissue.

Swollen tissue inside a cast must be attended to *immediately*. The cast has to be split to relieve the pressure, and the source of the swelling must be identified and corrected. Then a new cast is applied.

Sometimes swelling will cause neurologic symptoms because the tissue presses on nerves. Sometimes, however, there was neurologic damage at the time of the fracture, but it was not immediately diagnosed, and symptoms appeared some time after the cast was applied. Whatever the cause, the cast must be removed and the symptoms relieved. If this is not attended to at once, the person risks permanent neurologic damage. Again, doctors sometimes neglect to tell their patients what can happen, and the person has no way of knowing what's part of the normal healing process and what isn't.

The third principle is mostly a safety precaution, but it's important. If the bone fragments slip out of alignment, the wrist won't heal properly, and either the person will be left with a permanent deformity, or he or she will have to have the bone surgically broken and reset. Neither alternative is acceptable and can almost always be prevented by proper postoperative care.

In summary, the three principles of casting can be translated into direct action:

• If an above-the-knuckle cast has not been applied, insist on a shorter cast—or change doctors.

• Exercise the fingers enough so they remain fully flexible. Some pain now will prevent permanently "frozen" joints in the future. Singlehandedly crumpling a sheet of newspaper is a good exercise and should be repeated 15 times a day—five sheets three times a day.

• Get *immediate* attention (go to an emergency room if necessary) for swelling inside the cast and for sensations of numbness, tingling, or absence of sensation.

• Insist on periodic X-rays while the cast is on.

Pinning bones in place after a Colles fracture is a type of immobilization, used together with a plaster cast, when the fracture is particularly severe; for example, in a comminuted fracture, when most physicians use pinning routinely. Some doctors use pins only when the bone fragments have not begun to fuse two weeks after the original break.

The purpose of pinning is to hold the bone fragments together, much as nails hold two pieces of wood together. The pins are usually placed at the distal (near the hand) and proximal (near the elbow) ends of the radius, with the distal one going through one of the metacarpals (the small bones of the hand) as well. The end of the pin that protrudes from the skin is then embedded in the plaster cast, and the bone fragments are held rigidly in place.

Pinning is a surgical procedure in which the pins, which vary in size depending on the size of the bones and the nature of the break, are screwed or hammered into place. Some are less than a quarter of an inch thick, more like wire than nails, and some are as thick as large bolts. The pins are left in for six to eight weeks. One of the benefits of pinning is that a short cast (below the elbow) can be substituted for one that extends several inches above the elbow. This obviously leaves the elbow free, which can prevent problems later.

Pins can break, although this happens only rarely, and the hole through which it is inserted can become infected. Other than those, there are no medical drawbacks to the procedure. After the acute pain has disappeared, some people complain of a dull ache where the pins were hammered in, but this usually disappears in another week or so. The person can feel the pin, but it doesn't hurt and is easy to get used to.

The pin is removed when the fracture has healed (in the doctor's office without anesthesia), and a lighter cast or splint is applied for another week or so. Pin removal hurts—but only for the time of actual removal—from ten seconds to perhaps a minute. Then it's over, except for a residual ache that's gone the next day. Usually, there's a tremendous sense of relief at having the pins out.

There is some controversy about carrying the wounded hand around in a sling. True, a cast is heavy and awkward, but a sling discourages movement of the elbow and shoulder, which should be encouraged. There have also been cases of damage to the nerves in the back of the neck because of the constant weight of the cast. Some compromise between freedom of movement and relief from carrying the heavy burden can be worked out on the doctor's advice.

People with broken wrists should be encouraged, even advised, to do as much as they can with their affected arm and to do planned routine exercises for the fingers, elbow, and shoulder. Everything will take two or three times as long, of course, but it's better to struggle for 15 minutes hooking a brassiere than to leave muscles unused by asking someone else to do it. Care should be taken not to wet the cast, but this doesn't mean that one can't bathe. A plastic trash bag tucked into the ends of the cast will keep it dry.

Heppenstall says, "We do not routinely use a formalized physical therapy program following discontinuance of immobilization [removal of the pins and cast], but rely on active functional exercises. We reserve physical therapy for those patients with poor motivation who require constant supervision and encouragement."[4]

Elderly people are more likely to require formal physical therapy after the cast comes off than younger ones because they may be timid about exercising. They may have arthritis in other joints, and they may simply not be used to a regular exercise program. Also, some people with osteoporosis erroneously believe that exercise increases the chance of breaking a bone, and after the trauma of one fracture, they may fear another.

Even after the pins and cast are removed, there is a period of disability, the duration of which varies depending on age, the severity of the fracture, and the activities expected of the wrist. That is, it will take longer to be able to pick up a suitcase than it will to open a can of beer. In general, a healthy person will be able to resume full activity in about three or four months. An older person with osteoporosis can be partially disabled for twice that long. Even then, changes in barometric pressure or certain kinds of movements (such as turning a door knob or rotating the outstretched palm to receive coins) can remind the person for the rest of his or her life that that wrist was once broken.

Most people have some degree of deformity or loss of range of motion even after complete healing. This should not be severe, however, if the fracture was properly reduced, and it can be compensated for by learning to do some things with the other hand and by using the elbow and shoulder to perform some of the wrist's functions.

Of the three major types of fractures most common in osteoporotic people, a broken hip is the most disastrous because it has the most serious and long-lasting consequences. In fact, about 20 percent of all people who break their hips (usually elderly women) are dead within the first year, many within the first month. A full 50 percent never walk again, and many of these have no choice but to spend the rest of their lives in a nursing home.

However, things are improving. Says Heppenstall, ". . . early diagnosis and treatment are essential to improving survival rates. The trend in recent years has been, through early open reduction and early fixation,* to mobilize these patients as quickly as possible and so to avoid the disastrous complications of prolonged immobilization of these old people. This goal has been accomplished by innovative surgical procedures to obtain stability at the fracture site and improved technical design and quality of metallic devices for internal fixation. Although the patients are in a high-risk category owing to their advancing age and concomitant medical problems, several studies have revealed a definite decrease in the morbidity [illness] and mortality rate following aggressive surgical treatment. Results to date certainly justify the concept of early treatment and energetic physical therapy to return these patients to an active role in society."[5]

*Fixation is the joining of the two broken ends of the femur.

In other words, the sooner the hip is pinned and the person is up and moving around, the less likely he or she will be to die or be permanently disabled.

When we talk about a broken hip, we are really talking about breaking the neck of the femur (the long bone running from the knee to the pelvis) just below where the round "head" at the top of the femur (figure 8) fits into the socket in the pelvic bone. This is normally one of the strongest, most stable, and most flexible joints in the body, and it is surrounded and protected by some of the body's most highly developed muscles. Normally, it does a tremendous amount of the body's structural work without complaint. For example, when one stands on one leg, the amount of weight borne

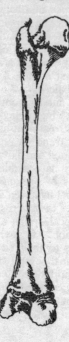

FIGURE #8
Femur Including Heads

by that hip is two and a half times body weight, and when one runs, the force placed on each hip during each stride is four and a half to five times body weight. The joint is so strong, in fact, that young people almost never break a hip except when it is subjected to excessive force, as, for example, during an automobile accident. However, older people break their hips easily because the neck of the femur is composed mostly of trabecular or spongy bone which is highly susceptible to osteoporosis.

About twice as many women as men break their hips, and as one would expect, the incidence of hip fracture increases with age. The fracture can occur anywhere in the neck of the femur (figure 9), but the three most common sites are: (1) high, almost at the base of the head of the bone, (2) straight across the middle, and (3) low, near the top of the shaft of the femur.

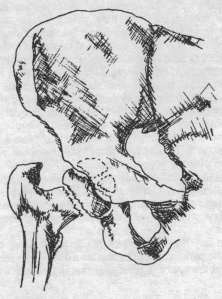

FIGURE #9
Fractured Head of Femur

The location of the fracture is not as important as the extent of the injury and the fact that, wherever the fracture line is, blood supply is almost always in danger of being cut off, as it indeed sometimes is. Loss of blood flow means that not only will the bone tissue itself start to die but that the fracture fragments can't heal. Blood supply must be quickly reestablished.

People with a broken hip are generally in great pain and can't bear weight. The fractured leg appears shorter than the other one because of its awkward position: rotated outward 30 or 40 degrees. Emergency treatment is mandatory.

The first thing the physician will do is take X-rays to determine the precise location and severity of the fracture. The next step is to operate on the hip, reduce the fracture, and place the pins. Hip pins also come in a wide variety, although as one would expect, they're bigger than wrist pins. Some of them look like screws with bolts on the end and some look like giant carpentry nails. If the array of orthopedic surgical instruments looks like a hardware store display, it seems only fitting because at times the orthopedic operating room sounds like a carpentry shop—complete with drilling, hammering, and sawing. Luckily, the patient is anesthetized and hears none of this.* Reducing a hip fracture is hard physical labor for the orthopedist, and if one watches such an operation, it's easy to see why the patient has so much postoperative pain. While the person is anesthetized, more X-rays are taken right in the operating room to make certain that the hip has been replaced in the correct position and that the pins are properly placed.

The most important consideration in healing, according to Heppenstall, is the reduction method. That is, the better the fracture is reduced and pinned, the more likely it is that it will heal completely and with as little postoperative deformity as possible.

The third step is to get the person moving again as soon as possible. The patient is kept in bed for a day or two following surgery, and a trapeze (a triangular metal grab bar which is

---

*If the person is very old and debilitated and general anesthesia would be too much of a risk, spinal anesthesia *might* be substituted.

suspended from an overhead frame) is hung over the head of the the bed so the patient can hold onto it to move around and hoist himself or herself on and off the bedpan. Unfortunately, some old people don't have the strength in their arms and chest to use the trapeze and are thus less able to move around and prevent postoperative complications. Using the trapeze is also more difficult for heavy people.

During the period of bed rest, a physical therapist should do what is called passive range of motion exercises; that is, putting each joint through its normal range of motion to prevent joint stiffening and loss of muscle tone, which happens amazingly quickly to a bedridden person, especially an elderly one.

On the second or third day after surgery the person can sit in a chair, and the next day he or she begins walking with the help of a walker, a metal "cage" on four legs that one holds onto for support and stability. Weight-bearing on the broken hip is increased gradually, and by the time the patient is discharged from the hospital (in about two weeks), he or she is up to almost full weight-bearing and may even have discarded the walker for crutches. X-rays are taken before the person leaves the hospital and again a month later.

During all this time, postoperative complications must be prevented. Pneumonia is the most frequent and deadly complication of hip fracture in the elderly. Heppenstall says that the prefracture physical state is directly related not only to the rate of healing but also to the rate of complications, and even to the death rate. Men die of broken hips about twice as often as do women, and the older the person the more likely they are to die or suffer serious complications.

Proper reduction of a broken hip, prevention of complications, and the subsequent gradual increase in physical activity—all must be done and supervised by a highly competent orthopedist. This can be a problem for someone with a broken hip who needs immediate treatment. Most elderly people, unless they have had other bone problems, do not know a competent orthopedist to call when they suddenly break a hip. What usually happens is that they are taken to the nearest emergency room and treated by the orthopedist there. If they are wealthy or have insurance or have the wherewithal themselves or are accompanied by a friend or relative, they can request a doctor of their own choice. They can also go to another hospital (and pay for the ambulance themselves) if the orthopedist they want is on staff there. And if the person with a broken hip is accompanied by someone, that someone can take the time and effort to make a few phone calls to get a recommendation for an orthopedist.

However, if the person is poor, on Medicare or Medicaid, unconscious, woozy from pain and shock, confused, or otherwise alone and vulnerable, an orthopedic resident will most likely do the surgery. This is not to imply that all residents are less than competent; in fact, some are better and more conscientious than physicians who have been practicing for years. It is to say, however, that they are almost always less experienced, and this means that they may or may not do as good a job as an experienced orthopedic surgeon. Because of the way hospitals (and the economic system on which they are based) are organized, there's not much one can do about this situation. This is not to say that everything will not turn out well. We include it here simply as a description of the way things are.

There are several late complications of hip fracture, some of them serious and debilitating. The most common is called avascular necrosis: the death and rotting away of bone tissue because it hasn't received enough blood. The best way to prevent this is by operating as soon as possible after the injury so that blood vessels can be reconnected. Also, proper reduction and pinning will prevent the blood vessels from tearing again after the surgery when weight-bearing begins.

Nonunion, that is, the refusal of the bone fragments to grow back together, occurs in from 10 to 45 percent of all broken hips. Excellent surgical technique can prevent some nonunion, but sometimes the bones are simply too old or too osteoporotic to make use of the best reduction technique in the world. If bones do not join eventually, there are two techniques that can be used: bone graft in the young and total hip replacement in the old.

The bone and/or joint can become infected. If the bone can be preserved—that is, if it hasn't been destroyed by the infectious process—the bacteria can often be killed by massive doses of antibiotics given both intravenously and directly into the site of the infection. The latter requires a complicated irrigation system that is painful and debilitating.

If the bone can't be saved or the infection routed, the hip must be replaced. Fortunately, this is rare.

Total hip replacement, the technical term for which is prosthetic replacement, has been done for many years, but the materials and techniques are continually being improved. The operation is simple to describe but complicated to do: the entire ball and socket joint is permanently replaced and cemented to healthy bone. It is often the only solution for elderly people with osteoporosis and in many cases has meant the difference between permanent crippling and a reasonably active life. The only two complications, both rare, are infection at the operative site and loosening of the prosthesis because the cement hasn't held. Infection can be controlled, and the new hip can be recemented, or even replaced, but this means another operation.

Broken bones hurt; in fact, bone pain can be excruciating. What makes a fracture bearable, however, even though it is painful, uncomfortable, handicapping, and a damn nuisance, is the fact that it is temporary. The cast will come off eventually; bones heal; pain recedes; and life eventually gets back to normal.

Sometimes, however (more often in older people than in younger ones), pain hangs around for longer than it should and becomes chronic. Chronic pain can be steady and unremitting, but more often it is intermittent and depends for its strength and intensity on a number of variables: physical activity and stress, general fatigue, the condition of the bones, diet, emotional factors, and even the weather.

The difference between chronic and acute pain is that the former has no foreseeable end, which is what makes it so unpleasant to live with and so difficult to treat. Most of the usual chemical methods of pain relief are not appropriate because of the problem of drug dependence. Thus, in addition to the pain itself, one has to cope with depression, demoralization, and hopelessness. Sometimes the pain is so ever-present and/or so severe (and the person's coping mechanisms so inadequate) that the pain becomes the central focus of existence, and life is effectively ruined.

Luckily, this is rare in both osteoporosis itself and in people who have had a fracture, but it does happen often enough to warrant some discussion and to offer some suggestions:

• The emotional response to chronic pain is as important as the pain itself. Even those who cope well in the beginning and take the pain in stride, eventually feel beaten down, and the pain is constantly in their thoughts. Before they are totally consumed by pain, they should be evaluated by one of the many pain control clinics around the country. It's easy to find a nearby one by calling the neurology department of the nearest large hospital or medical center.

• Because chronic pain eventually affects one's entire life, it also eventually affects family, friends, and co-workers. This is why pain control clinics include the family in whatever treatment is prescribed.

• Although no one *likes* pain, many people realize the manipulative uses of chronic pain and can soon turn the pain to their own psychological advantage. This is another reason why family is included in the treatment program.

• Chronic pain must be diagnosed in the same way that acute pain is. It may be that not all the pain is entirely chronic; that is, the original pain-producing medical problem may have given way to another problem that is at least partially correctable. The chronic pain sufferer should have a thorough diagnostic evaluation by doctors who will take the pain—and the sufferer—seriously.

• There are specific treatments for chronic pain, all of which should be prescribed and supervised by an appropriate physician (sometimes a neurologist, sometimes a psychiatrist, etc.), for example: surgery on nerve endings; chemical nerve block; electrical stimulators to interrupt the pain message to the brain; individual psychotherapy; group therapy; support groups; family therapy; occupational therapy; behavior modification; biofeedback; hypnosis; acupuncture; physical therapy; exercise; and medication.

• People with chronic pain can become desperate enough to fall victim to all kinds of quacks, charlatans, and purveyors of fake remedies, some of which can be exceedingly expensive, and some of which can be harmful. These should be avoided.

Chapter Five

DIET

*E*veryone seems to be diet-conscious these days, and older people are no exception. Not only do they care about calories and nutrients, they want to eat the best quality food for the least amount of money. With the ever-increasing cost of groceries and with more people living on the fixed income of a pension and/or Social Security, eating well without seriously straining one's budget is not always easy.

Everyone cares about calories; most elderly people are concerned about cholesterol and saturated fat (primarily that contained in food from animal rather than vegetable sources); and they should be concerned about calcium. This makes menu planning somewhat troublesome because the best (although not the only) sources of calcium are dairy products, which tend to be high in animal fat and calories. The next best source is very dark green leafy vegetables which are not always in season and are not always available in all supermarkets even when they are in season (though they may be available frozen). Nor does everyone like these highly flavored vegetables like broccoli, turnip greens, mustard greens, and kale. It appears, then, that a person who intends to take the full recommended 1500 mg a day of calcium will need to take some of that mineral in tablet form (unless he or she is willing and able to drink five glasses of milk—preferably skim or low-fat—each and every day, or to eat the equivalent amount of cheese or yogurt). The number of tablets will depend on how much natural calcium one gets each day. I shall describe later in the chapter how to calculate the number of tablets to take.

Many foods have some calcium but so little as to make them useless as reasonable sources of the mineral. For example, one would have to eat 29 apples or bananas, 15 carrots, 13 cups of orange juice, nine cups of strawberries, three pounds of butter, 73 cups of black coffee, two quarts of wine, ten eggs, and 97 frankfurters to get the calcium in a cup of milk. The thought of eating such amounts is either ludicrous, disgusting, or downright dumb (as in that much coffee, wine, or eggs every day). Some foods have no calcium at all, and some have enough so they can be used as effective sources of the mineral in menu planning. Space precludes a complete list of the calcium content of all foods, but those readers who want a complete list can find one in the many nutrition books available in bookstores and libraries or free from the government. The best and most complete information guide to all the nutrients in all foods is a pamphlet called "Nutritive Value of Foods: Home and Garden Bulletin Number 72." United States Department of Agriculture, 1981. It is available from the U.S. Government Printing Office, Washington, D.C. 20402.

There are, however, foods that are particularly excellent sources of calcium; in fact the following list contains the only foods that have sufficient amounts of the mineral (in the right-hand column in milligrams) to justify taking them into account while planning a menu. They are:

Whole milk	1 cup	290
Skim milk	1 cup	302*
Chocolate milk	1 cup	280
Buttermilk	1 cup	285
Light cream	1 tbsp	14
Sour cream	1 tbsp	14
Hot cocoa	1 cup	298
Plain low-fat yogurt	1 cup (8 oz)	245
Vanilla ice cream	1 cup	176
Sherbet	1 cup	102

---

*Some sources list whole milk and skim milk as having the same amount of calcium.

Cheddar cheese	1 oz	204*
Swiss cheese	1 oz	272
Processed American cheese	1 oz	174
Blue cheese	1 oz	150
Low-fat cottage cheese	1 cup	155
Grated Parmesan cheese	1 cup	1376
Skim milk ricotta cheese	1 cup	669
Egg	1	28
Homemade macaroni and cheese	1 cup	362
Sardines	1 oz	86
Salmon	3 oz	225
Bluefish	3 oz	244
Crabmeat	1 cup	246
Oysters	1 cup	343
Haddock	3 oz	210
Shad	3 oz	266
Shrimp	3 oz	224
Oil packed tuna, drained	3 oz	199
Lean broiled ground beef	3 oz	196
Lean roast beef	3 oz	158
Cabbage	1 cup	252
Okra	1 cup	194
Rhubarb	¾ cup	156
Broccoli	1 cup	176
Beet greens	1 cup	198
Collard greens	1 cup	304
Dandelion greens	1 cup	280
Kale	1 cup	268
Mustard greens	1 cup	376
Spinach	1 cup	196
Turnip greens	1 cup	378

Nutritional requirements for the elderly are not so different from those of younger people except in a few regards. We have already mentioned the need for extra calcium, and

---

*Other cheeses have as much or more calcium. The ones listed here are representative samples.

older people need fewer calories than younger ones because their metabolism slows down, and they are generally more sedentary than they were in their youth. However, the eating patterns of a lifetime are difficult to change, and it's probably best not to attempt it in later years. Rather, people with osteoporosis might consider modifying their eating habits slightly to conform to the requirements of the disease, a quieter lifestyle, and advancing age.

Regarding diminished calorie requirements, the National Center for Health Statistics says that a woman who weighs 120 pounds (55 kg) needs 1800 calories a day to maintain her weight at age 65, whereas she needed 2100 calories when she was twenty years younger. Three hundred calories is a piece of fudge cake, a small portion of steak, a slice of pizza "with everything on it," or pasta with lots of cream, cheese, and sausage instead of pasta with vegetables. Three hundred calories may also be simply larger quantities of the same food, or it may be the same amount of different food. And—300 calories a day is the difference between creeping pudginess and the maintenance of one's former weight.

A calorie is not a nutrient; it is a unit of heat analogous to a volt of electricity. One calorie is the amount of heat needed to raise the temperature of one kg of water one degree Centigrade. Calories are the fuel that converts food into energy, and without energy all body systems would run down. The more energy one expends, the more fuel (calories) is burned, and depending on the proportion of fuel intake and energy expenditure, a person will lose or gain weight. Thus, a calorie has no function except as fuel in the same way as electricity has no function except to make the machinery go and to make sound come out of the stereo. That is, the electricity that goes through the motor of a food processor does nothing for the processor. It doesn't improve it, repair it, reconstitute its plastic housing, and it certainly doesn't wash it! By the same token, calories do not repair damaged tissue or contribute to the formation of new tissue.

Nutrients are the substances that make possible all other body functions, and each nutrient has a different function. The major ones are:

- Proteins, the essential builders of tissue, are composed

of amino acids. They not only contribute to the formation of new tissue (for example, creating new bone to replace that which has been resorbed and forming new blood cells in reaction to a cut or to the natural death of existing blood cells), they also repair diseased or damaged tissue. Protein, for instance, is necessary to heal a bone fracture. Almost all foods contain some protein, but the proportion and quality vary widely depending on the number of amino acids the food protein contains. Fish, meat, eggs, and dairy products are complete proteins; that is, they contain a full complement of required amino acids, whereas vegetable proteins are incomplete because they lack one or more amino acids.

• Carbohydrates are sugar and starch which supply energy; in fact, about two-thirds of one's total caloric intake comes from carbohydrates. When a person eats too few carbohydrates, stored fat is broken down into its essential carbohydrate elements, which is what happens on a reducing diet. When body fat is completely used up, protein is broken down to supply energy. This is what happens when a person is starving. Carbohydrates are either simple or complex. Examples of the former are found in heavily sugared foods such as candy and pastry. Complex carbohydrates are found in rice, pasta, and grains.

• Fats, known technically as lipids, are a highly concentrated form of food energy and are required for the absorption and metabolism of Vitamins A, E, D, and K. Fat is stored under the skin and around certain organs such as the heart and liver to protect them. Fat helps regulate body temperature and protects underlying bones, muscles, and other tissues from injury.

Saturated fat is primarily animal fat, and unsaturated fat comes mostly from vegetable sources. At one time it was commonly believed that high levels of saturated fat in the diet contributed to an increased risk of cardiovascular disease. More recent research, however, has been unable to prove a direct cause-and-effect link between animal fat and heart attack and stroke, though there is no proof that one can eat an unlimited amount of animal fat with impunity. Until such time as there is direct evidence one way or another, and because fat contains such a high concentration of calories, it is probably best to adopt a "wait-and-see" attitude about the relationship between fat and cardiovascular disease—and to limit fat consumption.

• Fiber is not actually a nutrient, but it is important to the digestive process. It speeds up elimination and softens and adds bulk to the stool, which *may* help prevent colon cancer. Raw fruits and vegetables contain the highest fiber content and can help prevent constipation, but they also sometimes create gas and diarrhea.

• Vitamins are organic substances that have no calories and thus do not provide energy. They are, however, essential to good nutrition because they are the catalysts for certain chemical reactions. For example, Vitamin D aids in the absorption of calcium, and vitamin A converts fat into energy. If one eats a well-balanced diet, vitamin supplements (tablets) should not be necessary, but if one knows that he or she is not eating properly, one multivitamin tablet a day is a good idea.

As important as adequate vitamin intake is, over-vitaminization is equally harmful. More than ten times the recommended amount of any vitamin is called a megavitamin. For a variety of irrational reasons, many people believe that megavitamins are an appropriate antidote to real or imagined health problems, and they believe there is no such thing as taking too many vitamins. "Health nuts" tend to take megavitamins as do some fanatic exercisers. This is an incorrect and possibly dangerous practice; megavitamins *can* be too much of a good thing. For example, too much Vitamin C (the recommended dose is 60 mg a day) can cause diarrhea, kidney stones, and kidney damage. Too much Vitamin A (5000 International Units [IU] per day are enough) can cause headache, diarrhea, blurred vision, nervous system damage, and liver and bone damage. Vitamin A also contributes to bone loss. Vitamin D is particularly important to people with osteoporosis. Four hundred to 500 IU per day are recommended, but too much can cause headaches, weakness, nausea, blurred vision, and kidney and nervous system damage.

• Minerals are inorganic (chemical) substances such as calcium, sodium, phosphorus, potassium, and iron. Like vitamins, they do not provide calories for energy, and like vitamins they act as catalysts for chemical reactions. But they differ from vitamins in one important respect: they become part of the tissue itself, sometimes a major component. For example, calcium is integral to bones and teeth; without it they would literally fall apart.

All nutrients are important throughout all of life, but minerals, most especially calcium and phosphorus, should be of special interest to older people with osteoporosis. Phosphorus not only contributes to bone breakdown, it is also absorbed faster than calcium. For these reasons, most dietary experts recommend that elderly people consume about twice as much calcium as phosphorus. Foods that have a particularly poor calcium to phosphorus ratio (that is, far more phosphorus than calcium) are: bacon, liver, bran, chicken, red meat, corn, eggs, most fish, frankfurters and other processed meat, potatoes, pork, peanuts, peanut butter, and peas. This does not mean that people with osteoporosis should never eat foods that contain phosphorus; it means only that if they have eaten a particularly large quantity of phosphorus-rich foods, they should take extra calcium.

Herbs, roots, barks, spices, and all kinds of other flora have been ascribed with curative and restorative power over the centuries, and many of today's established drugs (such as quinine, digitalis, rauwolfia, and belladonna) are all found in naturally occurring vegetation. Herbs are rarely harmful and are sometimes beneficial if provided by an experienced herbalist, except when people depend on them to cure a disease or condition that requires something more. For example, catnip is fine for amusing one's feline friends, and some people even enjoy it brewed as a tea, but it is *not* a cure for cancer, kidney problems, or any other known ailment.

Some people believe that certain herbs can soothe some of the unpleasant effects of growing old. For example, if licorice root, sarsaparilla, elder, and ginseng are calming during the hot flashes of menopause, that's fine. And if people believe that chamomile or sage tea makes creaky joints feel looser, that's fine too. And if other things dug up in the woods can relax one to sleep, there's probably nothing wrong with that—except that *anything* taken to excess can be harmful. Many herbs have a potent medicinal effect, so potent in fact that pharmaceutical companies spend millions of dollars a year sending their scientists crashing about in various jungles to research these beneficial effects. Thus, one can take an overdose of a seemingly innocent and innocuous herb just as easily as one can take an overdose of seemingly innocent and innocuous aspirin, with the same disastrous effect. I *don't* mean to denigrate the use of herbs because many are obviously beneficial, but I *do* mean to give a warning about their use: do *not* use them as medicine or as a stopgap remedy for a symptom that could be the first indication of a serious medical problem.

Just as nutrition is crucially important to growing children, so is it essential for older people, albeit in a different way. Instead of counting on nutrients to aid in the growth and development of all body tissues, the elderly must depend on them to slow and minimize the deterioration of those tissues.

Each body system is characterized by particular signs of aging. The cardiovascular system (heart and blood vessels) is marked by a thickening and loss of elasticity of blood vessels. The heart itself remains the same size or shrinks slightly, but the valves can become less resilient and therefore function less efficiently. Since cardiovascular diseases are the leading cause of death of all adult Americans, many older people bring cardiovascular problems with them into old age. These problems affect them in that they tire more easily, their hearts take a longer time to recover from physical and psychic stress, and they are sometimes confused because their brain cells aren't receiving enough oxygen because blood flow is diminished as arteries narrow and sometimes block completely. All this can also cause hypertension (high blood pressure) which, if severe, can cause visual disturbances, headache, and possibly a stroke.

The brain gets smaller and lighter as individual cells die; there is simply less brain, just as there is less bone in osteoporosis. Central nervous system deterioration has a profound effect on old people's lives. Their memory becomes fuzzy but not in a uniform way; recent memory may be unreliable, but recollection of distant events is sharp. This produces the classic picture of an old person who can't remember what he or she ate for dinner last night but can describe in full detail an adolescent dance or flirtation. This quirk of memory tends to disconnect the elderly from the present and strengthen ties with the past.

The ability to conceptualize and solve complex problems is not significantly impaired, but sleep patterns change. The elderly tend to sleep less, and one wonders if there are not strong psychological components to this decreased amount of sleep: perhaps a reluctance to spend precious remaining time asleep or the fear that sleep may turn to death.

Central nervous system changes also can cause changes in gait, diminished reflexes, and decreased mobility. All this constitutes a safety hazard. An older person can't run from a mugger on the street or move fast out of the way of an onrushing car. He or she can become trapped in a burning building and is likely to be knocked down by crowds.

Musculoskeletal changes result from, in addition to osteoporosis, a general wasting of muscle tissue and loss of strength. Joints are not as loose and mobile as they used to be, tendons shrink; the older person is less supple and therefore less mobile.

Age affects the gastrointestinal system to widely varying degrees. Many people lose their teeth (due more often to gum disease than to cavities), and certain digestive processes slow, such as stretching of the esophagus and peristalsis, the wavelike movements of the digestive system that push the food along and through the various tubes. This is one of the reasons why the elderly eat less food at one time and need to take small bites.

Constipation is another common complaint. It is caused by the slowing of digestive processes, diminished physical activity, ingestion of less roughage because of decreased ability to chew, and the relatively high price of foods that tend to prevent constipation (fresh produce, whole grains, and meat).

Among the most disturbing changes of old age are those in the sensory functions, and sooner or later most of the senses dull. Vision dims because of cataracts, glaucoma, and the aging of retinal cells. Poor vision in the elderly is more than a nuisance; it can be a handicapping defect that leads to loneliness and isolation. Deafness is an even greater cause of isolation because if one can't hear, one can hardly communicate with others. Old age is not the best time to learn a new (sign) language, and hearing aids are only a partial solution.

Skin loses moisture and elasticity; loss of fat beneath the skin makes old people more sensitive to cold; and the wrinkling of skin and graying of hair can be psychologically depressing because it's "proof" that old age is inevitable. The size and strength of the American cosmetic industry indicates just how frightened we are of appearing old and how we will go to great lengths to prevent that.

Nothing can totally prevent all this deterioration, but adequate nutrition can hold it at bay for as long as possible. However, one of the major problems of the elderly obtaining good nutrition is money. Good food is expensive, and there's no getting away from the fact that it's more expensive to eat well than not. More elderly people starve to death in the United States (or die of diseases in which malnutrition is a strong contributory factor) than any other single age group. The myth that the elderly can live on less money than younger people is just that: a myth. Food, clothing, transportation, and housing are not subject to "senior citizens" discounts, and health care is only slightly less expensive. If elderly people live on less money, it's because many of them are forced to subsist on only the bare necessities. The American dream of a comfortable and relaxed retirement filled with books, travel, and entertainment has been turned into a nightmare by inflation for all but the minority of those who are wealthy enough to live on more than the average fixed income.

Nutrition seems to be one part of life that is most affected by age and poverty. Elderly people's diets tend to be inadequate in both quality and quantity. Both problems are caused mainly by shortage of money, although they are aggravated by diminished appetite, poor cooking facilities, and chronic illness and fatigue that make cooking too much of a chore. Many older people are overweight (which tends to complicate cardiovascular and musculoskeletal problems) for a variety of reasons: poor eating habits that don't change as calorie requirements decrease; boredom, frustration, and loneliness that sometimes lead to eating as "something to do"; and overconsumption of high carbohydrate foods such as potatoes, rice, pasta, and junk food that tend to be less expensive and more filling than foods with high concentrations of proteins, vitamins, and minerals.

There are things that can be done about this. Medicare, officially known as Title XVIII of the Social Security Act, "Health Insurance for the Aged and Disabled," provides nutritional services, and one of the provisions of the Older Americans Act is one hot meal a day to be served to the aged, either in community centers or at home through such agencies as Meals on Wheels. These are federal mandates and are administered through state or community social service agencies.

One of the most important components of food and eating is the socialization of eating with people. It's boring and depressing to have to eat alone all the time, to cook for only one, to have no one to exclaim with over the deliciousness of the meal, and no one to chat with while the dishes are being washed. Eating communal meals or living in a communal house can alleviate isolation, and it can cut costs. In addition to the obvious social, emotional, and financial benefits of such an arrangement, the responsibility and pleasure of cooking for others almost guarantees well-balanced and enjoyable meals. Those who would tend to live on cold sandwiches and junk food because they did not have the energy and inclination to cook for themselves would be encouraged by their housemates or meal-mates to eat healthfully.

A way to encourage communal cooking and eating without communal living is for a number of elderly people in a neighborhood to form a "cooking cooperative" in which they come together for one or two meals a day. Yet another arrangement is to take meals at a local community center. The point in sharing meals is that everyone, regardless of cultural background, associates eating with socializing, and although a solitary meal while reading or watching television is often pleasurable, having to eat alone all the time is depressing, lonely, and demoralizing. Communal eating can be an appetite stimulant.

There are four basic food groups: the milk and dairy group which supplies calcium, high quality protein, and Vitamins A, B, and D; the meat and egg group which provides protein, iron, and some forms of Vitamin B; the fruit and vegetable group which supplies roughage, carbohydrates, Vitamins A, C, and others, and minerals; and the bread and cereal group which supplies carbohydrates, Vitamin B, iron, and other minerals. The Food and Nutrition Board of the National Academy of Sciences recommends that everyone eat four or more servings each day of the milk and dairy group, two or more servings of the meat and egg group, four servings of the fruit and vegetable group, and four servings of the bread and cereal group. A serving size varies as do the choices one can make from each group. If one is counting calories as well as milligrams of calcium, a person planning menus may need a calculator in addition to a pencil and paper when reading the cookbook and making out a grocery list.

Following are samples of foods from each group, the average serving size, and the number of calories:

MILK AND DAIRY GROUP

Whole milk	1 cup	160
Buttermilk	1 cup	90
Skim milk	1 cup	90
Cheddar cheese	1 oz	105
Ice cream	1 cup	300
Ice milk	1 cup	260
Dry milk powder	¼ cup	63
Cottage cheese	1 cup	240

MEAT AND EGG GROUP

Lean broiled ground beef	3 oz	245
Broiled chicken	3 oz	115
Baked lamb	3 oz	210
Fried liver	3 oz	195
Peanut butter	1 tbsp	100
Dried kidney beans	1 cup	230
Egg scrambled with milk and fat	1	110
Egg	1	75
Broiled fish	3 oz	135

FRUIT AND VEGETABLE GROUP

Baked potato	1 medium	90
Broccoli	1 cup	40
Cole slaw	1 cup	120
Peas	1 cup	115
Raw apple	1	70
Raw banana	1	85
Raw orange	1	60
Orange juice	1 cup	110

BREAD AND CEREAL GROUP

White bread	1 slice	65
Whole wheat bread	1 slice	56
Rye bread	1 slice	55
Plain muffin	1 average	118
Cooked macaroni	½ cup	85
Cooked rice	½ cup	93
Cooked spaghetti	½ cup	78
Cooked oatmeal	½ cup	65
Corn flakes	1 oz	110
Granola cereal	½ cup	195

Following is a list of the basic necessary nutrients and some foods that are a rich source of those nutrients:

Protein—milk, cheese, eggs, meat, grains, breads, cereals, legumes, nuts.

Calcium—dairy products, whole or enriched grains, green leafy vegetables.

Phosphorus—milk, cheese, lean meats.

Iron—organ meat (especially liver), egg yolk, green leafy vegetables, dried fruit, enriched grains.

Iodine—seafood, iodized salt.

Magnesium—whole grains, nuts, soybeans, dried beans and peas, cocoa, seafood.

Vitamin A—whole milk, cream, butter, liver, egg yolk, dark green or deep yellow vegetables or fruit, fortified margarine.

Vitamin C—citrus fruits, papaya, strawberries, melon, broccoli, potato, tomato, cabbage, green or chili peppers.

Folic acid—liver, dark green vegetables, dried beans, lentils, nuts.

Vitamin D—fortified milk, fortified margarine.

Vitamin E—vegetable oils, leafy vegetables, cereals, meat, eggs, milk.

Niacin—meat, peanuts, beans, peas, enriched grains.

Riboflavin—milk, liver, enriched grains.

Thiamine—pork, beef, liver, whole or enriched grains, legumes.

Vitamin B$_6$—wheat, corn, liver, meat.

Vitamin B$_{12}$—milk, eggs, meat, liver, cheese.

Folic acid and riboflavin don't sound like very appetizing things to eat, but chopped chicken liver (with lots of onion), a spinach or cheese omelet, a milkshake, a grilled cheese sandwich on rye probably do. Although one could get many nutrients (with the notable exception of protein, carbohydrates, and fats) from commercial vitamin tablets, people prefer to get them from the food they eat. And if one is going to eat, one might as well eat healthily as well as deliciously.

In the sample menus that follow we have given the *approximate* number of calories and milligrams of calcium from food and then the milligrams of calcium that must also be taken in tablet form based on a total recommended calcium intake of 1500 mg a day. Some of the meals are more balanced and complete than others, and some might even be downright unhealthy, but we have tried to be realistic. That is, people *do* grab pizza and soda for lunch or run out of the house in the morning munching on a toaster pastry.

DAY ONE

BREAKFAST
1 cup orange juice
Cereal, hot or cold, with 1 cup skim milk
Coffee

LUNCH
Swiss cheese sandwich on rye bread
½ cup cole slaw
1 cup skim milk

DINNER
6 oz steak
Baked potato with butter
1 cup spinach
2 glasses white wine
1 cup vanilla ice cream

Total calories—2278
Total calcium—2308

DAY TWO

BREAKFAST
1 cup grapefruit juice
Cheddar cheese omelet
Coffee

LUNCH
Spinach salad with hard boiled egg
Tea

DINNER
6 oz baked haddock
Scalloped potatoes
Broiled tomato
Apple pie
Coffee

Total calories—1809
Total calcium—1491

DAY THREE

BREAKFAST
½ cantaloupe
2 granola bars
Coffee

LUNCH
1 glass sherry
Fillet of sole meunière
Fresh asparagus
2 rolls with butter
Chocolate mousse

DINNER
1 low-calorie frozen fish dinner
Coffee

Total calories—1930
Total calcium—690
Extra calcium required—800

DAY FOUR

BREAKFAST
1 cup orange juice
2 scrambled eggs
3 sausage links
English muffin with butter
Coffee

LUNCH
Coffee
Danish pastry

DINNER
Shrimp sauteed with snow peas and apples
Tossed salad with sour cream dressing
1 glass white wine
2 peaches

Total calories—1800
Total calcium—370
Extra calcium required—1130

DAY FIVE

BREAKFAST
Fresh strawberries with sour cream
Cereal with 1 cup skim milk
Coffee

LUNCH
Cold fried chicken
2 ears corn on the cob
½ cup potato salad
Iced tea
Chocolate cake
Watermelon

DINNER
Cold cream of avocado soup
Tossed salad with dressing
Diet soda

Total calories—1680
Total calcium—850
Extra calcium required—650

DAY SIX

BREAKFAST
1 orange
Grilled American cheese sandwich
Coffee

LUNCH
Lemon yogurt
2 granola bars
Coffee

DINNER
Cream of tomato soup (made with milk)
Crab imperial
Broccoli
Tossed salad with dressing
1 glass white wine
Butterscotch pudding
Tea

Total calories—2100
Total calcium—1100
Extra calcium required—400

DAY SEVEN

BREAKFAST
1 cup orange juice
1 cup skim milk
2 toaster pop tarts

LUNCH
Sardine sandwich on whole wheat with mayonnaise
Ice cream bar
Coffee

DINNER
Baked pork chops with sweet potatoes
Tossed salad with blue cheese dressing
1 glass red wine
Stewed rhubarb with strawberries
Coffee

Total calories—1927
Total calcium—1000
Extra calcium required—500

DAY EIGHT

BREAKFAST
1 cup cottage cheese
2 pieces dry rye toast
Coffee

LUNCH
1½ cups macaroni and cheese
Diet soda

DINNER
2 cups chili con carne
Tossed salad with dressing
1 piece corn bread
2 glasses red wine
Banana cake
Coffee

Total calories—1960
Total calcium—775
Extra calcium required—750

DAY NINE

BREAKFAST
½ grapefruit
1 cup hot cream of wheat with 1 sliced banana and ½
    cup skim milk
Coffee

LUNCH
2 slices pizza with pepperoni
Diet soda

DINNER
Cabbage stuffed with sausage and tomato
Noodle pudding
Braised carrots
Apple pie
Tea

Total calories—1840
Total calcium—400
Extra calcium required—1100

DAY TEN

BRUNCH
Champagne with orange slices
Chicken and mushroom crepes with Mornay sauce
Banana nut bread
White wine
Lemon meringue pie
Coffee

DINNER
Grilled cheese sandwich with tomato
Broccoli
Apple
Coffee

Total calories—1725
Total calcium—1200
Extra calcium required—300

_____ *Chapter Six* _____

EXERCISE

_____

*A*n elderly person who has been sedentary most of his or her life should think about getting up to exercise, but the exercise program should begin the way porcupines make love—very, very carefully. The first thing is to have a complete physical examination. Cardiac stress tests have become popular recently, especially for people embarking on an exercise program after having been sedentary for a long time, but not all physicians believe this is necessary except under certain circumstances. Some of these might be hypertension, a high cholesterol level, personal or family history of heart attack, chest pain on exertion, diabetes, a resting heart rate of more than 80 beats a minute, taking longer than usual to get back to a resting heart rate after exertion, and shortness of breath with even mild exertion.

Jogging, even though it is very popular now, is not a good idea for people who have not exercised on a regular basis, as the risk of injury is far too great in such a strenuous weight-bearing exercise. Far better are brisk walking, swimming, stationary bicycling, and aerobic dancing. The irony is, however, that weight-bearing exercise is better for preventing and retarding osteoporosis than activity that does not put stress on the skeleton. The best thing is to have begun running, playing tennis, racquetball, squash, and the like in one's youth, but for people who are no longer young and who want to prevent the worsening of osteoporosis, a good compromise is brisk walking. There is some weight-bearing but not the kind of jarring stress on bones that significantly increases the risk of injury.

Brisk walking improves the condition of the cardiovascular system as it burns up calories and improves muscle tone. To derive cardiovascular benefits, one must exercise three to five times a week at a sustained heart rate of 110 to 120 beats a minute for 15 to 60 continuous minutes. Exercise for longer than that will burn up more calories, but it won't improve cardiovascular fitness.

The most convenient pulses are the radial in the wrist and the carotid in the neck. On most, the radial can be felt just below the fleshy pad at the base of the thumb where the radial artery is close to the surface. The carotid artery runs along the side of the neck and is palpable an inch or so below the earlobe just beneath the jawbone. If one feels around gently with the first two fingers (*not* the thumb), there should be no trouble finding the pulse.

There are two kinds of muscle contractions into which all types of exercise fall: isotonic and isometric. The isotonic contraction involves moving a muscle so that it changes in length as the joint is moved; that is, when one bends one's elbow, the length of the muscles in both the forearm and the upper arm change. This is also called dynamic exercise, the most important element of which is the rhythmic contraction and relaxation of muscles. The effect is to enhance blood flow, thus constantly replenishing the supply of oxygen in the muscle tissue. Walking, bicycling, swimming, and all sports that involve running are examples of isotonic exercise. So are those done with the aid of exercise machines.

Isometric muscle contractions do not arise from joint movement; hence, the muscle length does not change. Isometric, also called static, exercise also increases blood flow because the muscles are contracted but not to the extent they are in isotonic exercise. An example of isometric exercise is weightlifting.

There are specific physiologic advantages to exercise, aside from the obvious psychologic and social ones:

• More blood, and thus more oxygen, is circulated to all body cells. In general, the better the blood supply, the healthier the cell.

• Cardiac output is increased; that is, the heart becomes more efficient, moving more blood with each beat of the pump. As the person continues to exercise regularly, the heart actually increases in size slightly, and this sustains the increased cardiac output.

• Vital capacity of the lungs (the amount of air they can hold) doesn't change much as a result of exercise, but breathing becomes progressively easier. However, long-term exposure to airborne pollutants (as in regular walking or running outdoors or playing tennis near a heavily traveled road) may be toxic.

• Lean tissue increases in proportion to the amount of fat tissue, and bone mass increases.

When doing any exercise, a warm-up and cool-down period is a good idea to prevent muscle cramps and injury. The idea of the warm-up and cool-down is to use the same muscles slowly that will be used quickly during the actual exercise. For example, if the exercise is to be brisk walking, the person should start out by walking slowly for five minutes before exercising, and afterward he or she should walk slowly again until the heart rate returns to almost the resting state.

Stretching before exercise is controversial because in older people the muscles are less elastic and stretch easily only when they are warm. Stretching cold muscles risks injuring them.

People exercise for three basic reasons: to improve muscle tone in order to look better, to increase cardiovascular efficiency for a longer life, and to burn calories. The last is the most easily controlled and measured; that is, the rate of "calorie burn" can be tailored to the amount of food eaten. In other words, one can do a specific exercise for a certain amount of time to counteract the extra calories in a piece of chocolate cake or hot fudge sundae. Following are some selections from the President's Council on Physical Fitness and Sports (1980) table of exercise to calorie burn ratio:

• Gardening—5 calories per minute
• Golf—4 calories per minute
• Walking upstairs—10 to 18 calories per minute
• Bowling—7 calories per minute
• Tennis—7 to 11 calories per minute

- Handball—7 to 11 calories per minute
- Cross country skiing—9 to 17 calories per minute
- Swimming—6.5 calories per minute
- Running at 5 mph—10 calories per minute
- Walking at 2 mph—6 calories per minute
- Reading, watching television, etc.—1.5 calories per minute
- Doing dishes, slow walking—2 calories per minute
- Active sex—13 calories per minute

It's nice to know that sex is even better than tennis for burning calories even though it's hard to believe that something generally done lying down is more strenuous than that done upright!

Whatever the exercise and whatever the surroundings in which it takes place, there are certain universal guidelines that apply. Whether one works out in an expensive gym wearing designer clothes or takes long walks in the neighborhood wearing old jeans and a college sweatshirt, one needs to be aware of certain safety principles:

- Be certain that the exercise will not aggravate an existing health problem. Only your doctor can advise you about that.

- Begin slowly and gradually work up to a full level of exercise. For example, if an exercise should be done ten times in a row, start with one or two times and gradually increase the number over the course of a week or so.

- Do not exercise to the point of exhaustion. Remember, this isn't the Olympics, and you aren't 18 years old. The ultimate purpose of exercise is to feel better, not to be so wiped out that you can't do anything else for the rest of the day.

- Never exercise immediately after a meal or after drinking alcohol when blood is drawn away from the periphery of the body (where it is most needed during exercise) toward the internal organs to aid in digestion.

- If you feel sick, dizzy, or weak while exercising, stop *immediately*.

- Drink lots of water after exercise. The more you sweat, the more you need to drink. There is some controversy about the value of commercially prepared drinks, such as Gatorade, that are supposed to replace lost electrolytes (trace elements and minerals). You're probably better off sticking to plain cool water. Ice water on a very hot stomach can cause nausea and vomiting. Dehydration, a dangerous condition sometimes severe enough to require hospitalization, especially in older people, can occur without warning, particularly in hot, humid weather.

• During summer or in hot climates, exercise in early morning or late afternoon to prevent heatstroke, which is serious and in rare cases can be fatal.

• When exercising in the sun, always wear a hat to prevent sunstroke.

• If you exercise outdoors in winter, take a long time for both warm-up and cool-down. The former is necessary to warm cold muscles, and the latter will prevent frostbite if you have worked up a sweat. If it is very cold, wear a loose-knit scarf and cover your mouth with it to warm the air before it enters your lungs.

• Use common sense. If you are exhausted, stop. If you don't feel well, don't start. Exercise is not a punishment.

• Concentrate on breathing as slowly and regularly as possible. Holding one's breath during strenuous exercise is a natural tendency, but this only increases the pressure within the chest and abdomen and puts unnecessary added stress on the heart.

• Don't walk or do other exercises in strong wind; this too creates unnecessary stress that doesn't burn additional calories and doesn't increase cardiovascular efficiency.

There are dozens of exercise and fitness books on the market that prescribe specific exercise programs for specific needs. What I provide here is an overview of the kinds of exercises that older people in general and those with osteoporosis in particular may find useful and practical.

The first set of exercises will improve sphincter control in the anus and around the urethra. A sphincter is a circular muscle that contracts and expands, sometimes voluntarily (as in the anal sphincter) and sometimes involuntarily (as in the muscles around the eyes). Some older people tend to have less sphincter control, especially some menopausal women who suffer from pelvic relaxation, the condition in which the bladder, rectum, uterus, and/or cervix tend to drop a little because the muscles and ligaments that support them are less effective than they used to be. These exercises should be done three or four times every hour:

- Tighten the anal sphincter as if to stop the passage of feces or gas.
- Tighten the vaginal/urethral muscles as if to stop the flow of urine.

Elderly people, especially if they have not exercised regularly, often have low back pain, and osteoporosis sooner or later will cause back pain. Following are some exercises that strengthen the back muscles. Each one should be done at least five times a week with five to ten repetitions while the person is lying on his or her back on a firm surface such as an exercise mat or thick carpet on the floor.

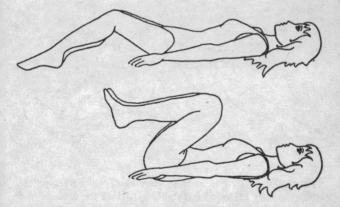

- *Figure 10:* **Lie flat with your legs bent; bring both knees as close to your chest as possible. Hold for a count of 5. Slowly return to the starting position.**

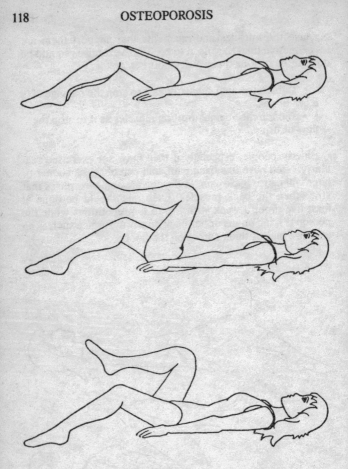

• *Figure 11:* **Bring one knee to your chest while keeping the other leg fully extended (straight out). Hold for a count of 5 and return to the starting position. Change legs, and repeat.**

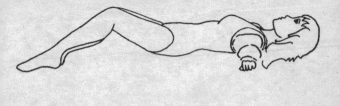

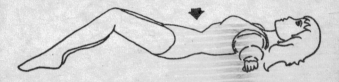

• *Figure 12:* Bend your knees while keeping your feet flat on the floor. Press the small of your back against the floor by contracting your buttocks and abdominal muscles. Hold for a count of 5.

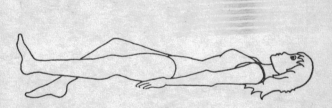

• *Figure 13:* Bend one leg and keep that foot flat on the floor. Raise the other leg 12 inches off the floor while keeping it straight. Hold for a count of 3. Lower the leg as slowly as possible. Change legs, and repeat.

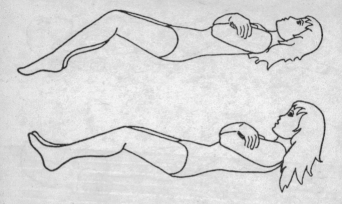

• *Figure 14:* Bend your knees and keep your feet flat on the floor; fold your arms across your chest. Then raise your head and shoulders, and hold for a count of 3. Roll down slowly.

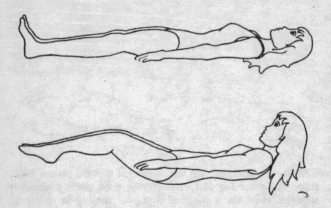

• *Figure 15:* Extend your legs straight out, keep your arms flat at your sides, and then raise your head and shoulders. Hold for a count of 3. Roll down slowly.

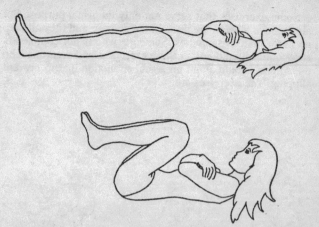

• *Figure 16:* Extend your legs and fold your arms across your chest. Bring both legs as close to your chest as possible. Return them slowly to the extended position, but do not let your ankles touch the floor. Hold for a count of 3. Relax.

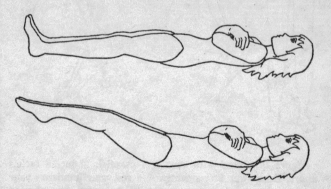

• *Figure 17:* Extend your legs and fold your arms across your chest. Raise your legs 12 inches off the floor, hold for a count of 3, and then slowly lower your legs.

Some exercises that serve not only the usual purpose but also relieve tension are done in the shower, and they all take no more than five minutes. Someone who is not completely sure-footed should *not* try these exercises, and everyone who does them should stand on a rubber suction mat to prevent slipping. The exercises are:

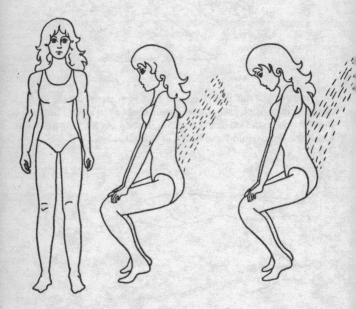

• *Figure 18:* **Stand with your feet parallel, about 18 inches apart. Bend your knees gently, and rest your hands on your thighs. The shower spray should hit the lower part of your back. Alternate pushing up on and "caving in" your back by raising and lowering your buttocks and tucking your head under and extending your neck. Repeat 5 times.**

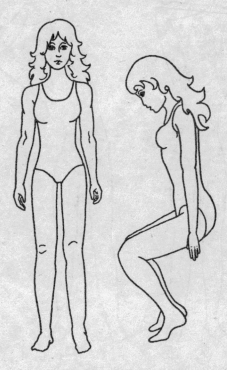

• *Figure 19:* For a total back stretch, stand straight, feet about 18 inches apart. As you exhale, slowly roll your body down by lowering your buttocks and bending your hips, knees, and ankles. Lower your body as far as it's comfortable and let your arms and head dangle. Then, as you inhale, slowly roll back up, using the muscles in your thighs and abdomen to raise you. Repeat 5 times.

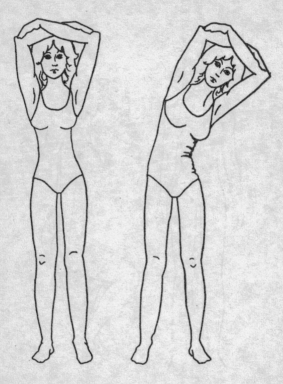

• *Figure 20:* Stand erect with feet firmly planted about 12 inches apart. Clasp your forearms or elbows over your head while pressing your shoulders down. As you exhale, stretch your upper body to the right, keeping your hips and waist still. As you inhale, return to center. Then do the same thing turning to the left. Repeat each pair 5 times.

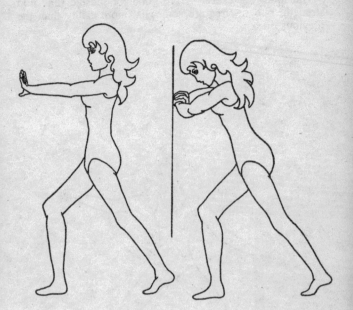

• *Figure 21:* Stand with your right leg bent forward and your left leg straight out behind you. Your feet should be about 30 inches apart. Place your arms straight out in front of you, and at shoulder height put your hands against the wall. Slowly lower your body toward the wall, bending your elbows and keeping your left leg straight, with both feet flat on the mat. Hold until you feel the stretch in the back of your calf. Push back to your original position. Repeat 5 times, then switch sides and repeat 5 more times.

The following exercises are good for muscle tone and strength, but they require somewhat more agility than the previous ones.

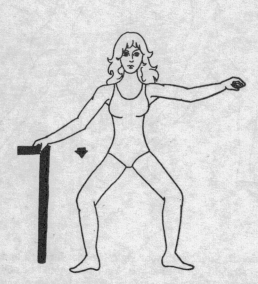

• *Figure 22:* Stand next to a piece of sturdy hip-height furniture such as a dresser or a club chair. Hold on with the right hand and extend your left arm straight out at shoulder height. Place your heels together with your toes pointed in opposite directions. Bend your knees while lowering your left arm with elbow bent. Hold for a count of 3. Slowly straighten your knees

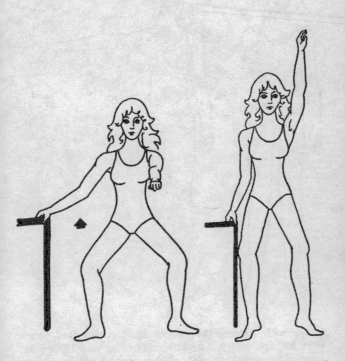

while extending your left arm, elbow bent in front of you. Hold for a count of 3. Slowly raise yourself on tiptoes (not so high that you lose your balance) while raising your left arm over your head. Hold for a count of three and slowly return to your original position. Repeat 5 times.

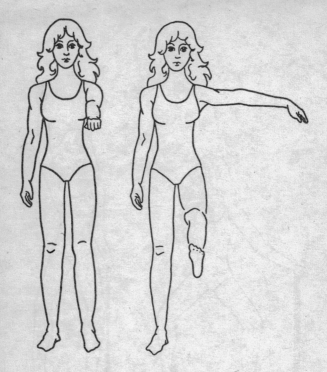

• *Figure 23:* Assume the starting position described above. With left arm raised straight ahead, swing your left leg forward as far as you can while moving your left arm behind you as far as you can, straight out at shoulder height. Hold for a count of 3. Slowly swing your left leg back and your left arm forward. Hold for a count of 3. Repeat 5 times, then turn around and do the arm and leg on the right side. Repeat 5 times.

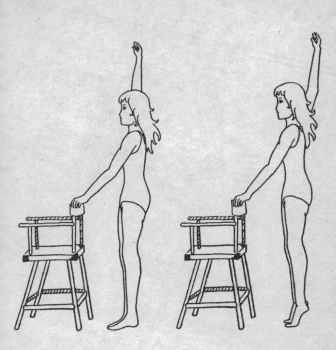

• *Figure 24:* Stand behind the chair with your left hand holding the chair back and your right arm straight overhead. Stand on tiptoe and at the same time stretch your right arm as far backward as it will comfortably go. Repeat 5 times. Switch sides and repeat 5 times.

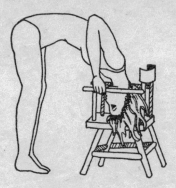

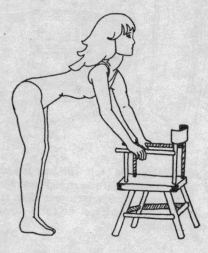

• *Figure 25:* Stand 2 feet in front of the chair and grasp its arms. Drop your head and chest into a deep forward bending position. Swing upward, raising your head and arching your body while leaning forward. Return to the starting position and repeat 4 times.

The following exercises are done lying on a flat surface and are good for the trunk, abdomen, and lower back:

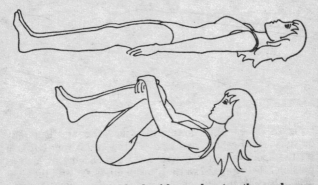

• *Figure 26:* Lie on your back with your legs together and arms at your sides. Grasp your right knee with both hands and pull the knee toward your chin. Raise your head and shoulders off the floor. Return to the starting position and repeat 8 times with each leg.

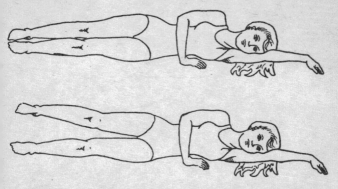

• *Figure 27:* Lie on your left side with your back straight and your right hand on the floor at waist level for balance. Raise your right leg as far as possible, keeping your knees straight. Lower your leg to the starting position. Repeat 5 times, then switch to the other side and repeat 5 more times.

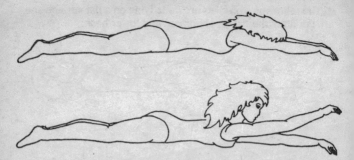

• *Figure 28:* Lie face down with your arms and legs fully outstretched. Keeping your elbows straight, lift your left arm off the floor while lifting your head and looking as high as possible. Return to the starting position. Repeat with the right arm. Alternate the arms and repeat the pairs 10 times.

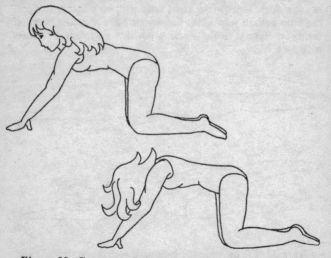

• *Figure 29:* Get onto all fours in the kneeling position with elbows straight, head up, and feet back. Arch your back upward by tensing your abdominal muscles. Lower your head and exhale hard. Hold for a count of 3 and return to the starting position. Repeat 4 times.

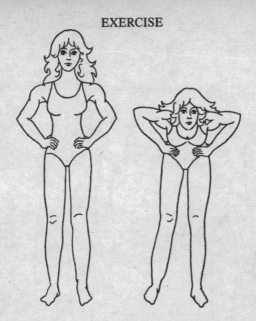

• *Figure 30:* Stand erect with feet about 24 inches apart and hands on hips. Slowly bend forward to a 90 degree angle. Hold for a count of 3 and return to the upright position. Repeat 10 times.

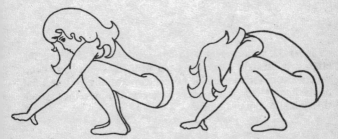

• *Figure 31:* Get onto all fours in a crouched position with your head down and arms outstretched. Slowly rock back until your buttocks touch your heels. Your elbows should bend and your back should curve into a rounded position. Repeat 5 times.

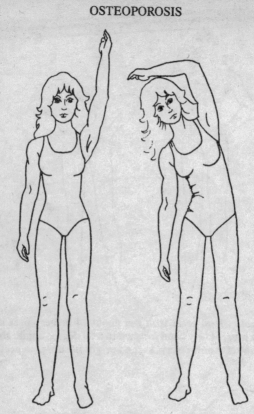

• *Figure 32:* Stand erect with one arm at your side and the other arm straight over your head with elbow straight. Bend your waist as far to one side as you can, keeping both feet flat on the floor. Hold for a count of 3. Repeat 10 times, then switch sides and do 10 more times.

Chapter Seven

INTERVIEWS

*R*oz Turner, 67, has the "classic" body shape of a victim of osteoporosis, short and small-boned, thin, almost no indentation at the waist, and a pronounced hump on her upper back.

She says she's had the hump (kyphosis) ever since she was a young girl, but it has become more severe with the osteoporosis. "I grew up in the Depression, and we didn't have much money for medical care. I don't think my parents could have afforded any correction even if we had been aware of such things. Before I was married, the doctor thought he could correct it [the hump], so he put me in one of those canvas braces which just about killed me. I couldn't stand it for more than a couple of hours at a time, and of course it didn't do a bit of good because I had such a severe curvature already."

Although Roz is the only one in her family who had kyphosis when she was a little girl, her mother and two sisters also fell victim to osteoporosis.

Roz first began noticing changes in the shape of her body over a decade ago when she was about four years past menopause. She once asked her husband, John, to measure her and was shocked at the result. "I found that I'd lost two inches, and I thought I'd better lose some more weight because now I was too heavy according to those insurance height-weight charts. So I lost 15 pounds and went on my way."

Then she noticed that her waist had started to thicken.

"The waistbands of clothes that had fitted me for years were too tight. I wasn't prepared for that. I don't think most women are prepared for the way their bodies change."

At around this time her lifestyle changed too. She quit her job as an elementary schoolteacher and began working as a secretary. "When I was a teacher, I was on my feet running around all day. Then I just sat for eight hours. I think that might have had something to do with it."

Roz went through menopause when she was 52, but just one month ago she began to take replacement estrogens. "My doctor was afraid of the risk of cancer, but he decided that the osteoporosis was becoming so severe that I really needed it. The bottom line was a productive life. He didn't want me to become a cripple or to break a hip." So she decided she would rather risk endometrial cancer (which is a very low risk) than a worsening of the osteoporosis.

The kitchen table is littered with pill bottles, most of which belong to her husband, who has severe asthma. But Roz's medicine is there too. Her gynecologist prescribed calcium supplements, but she had no idea how much of the mineral is in each tablet. The bottle had one of those little pharmacy labels on it as well as the manufacturer's label. The calcium she is taking is readily available over the counter without a prescription, but she was having the pharmacist "fill" the doctor's prescription—and paying about three times as much as she had to.

When she was shown that each tablet contains only 270 mg, she said, "Oh my, I had no idea." Neither did she have an idea of how much calcium she *should* be taking. Her gynecologist said to take one tablet a day, so on his recommendation she was missing about 80 percent of required calcium. To make matters worse, she hates milk and eats little cheese and no yogurt.

Not only is Roz taking far too little calcium, she's paying far too much for what she *is* taking because neither her gynecologist nor the pharmacist ever told her that not only doesn't she need a prescription for calcium, but there are far cheaper brands that are equally good. Moreover, she was overdosing on Vitamin D, taking over 15,000 units a day. The recommended amount is 400 units a day. Her gynecologist prescribed 100,000 units a week, and she didn't know that she was already getting 800 units a day in the two multivitamins she took every morning.

Why did her doctor prescribe so much Vitamin D?

"I don't know. I'll have to ask him."

Did she ever read the label to find out what and how much of everything is in the multivitamins she takes every day?

"No, I had no idea there were all those good things in there." She had never asked her doctor to explain anything about any medication, but she said she would surely find out now.

When she did, the doctor apologized profusely for the mistake and straightened out the dosages.

Osteoporosis has changed Roz's life as well as the shape of her body. "You know, I used to carry the Hoover up and down the stairs and just swing it around to wherever I needed it. But I realized that I could snap my hip just like that and really be out of commission. And another thing: I read in a magazine article that women with osteoporosis shouldn't make beds and lift the mattress. I'd been doing that without giving it a thought, but I've stopped now because I'm afraid of breaking my back."

One of Roz's sisters is severely handicapped by osteoporosis, and Roz envisions that sort of life for herself if she isn't careful. "She can't even lift a casserole to put it in the oven. She can hardly lift the teakettle unless there's practically no water in it. It can really change your life."

Roz is now extremely careful not to fall and always holds the banister when she goes up and down stairs. She's had two cataract operations and is a little insecure about her eyesight, so that slows her progress even more. "I guess people get impatient with me, but I've decided to go slowly and be really careful."

She has no pain even though she once had a hairline ankle fracture as a result of walking around for several hours on too-high heels. At the time that happened she had a complete bone scan which was when her Paget's disease was discovered. Paget's is chronic inflammation of the bones that tends to thicken and distort them.* It has nothing to do with

---

*It should not be confused with Paget's disease of the breast, which is something else entirely.

osteoporosis and is symptomless, but it *is* there and *may* also have contributed to her changing body shape.

Roz was wearing a bedroom slipper because she had broken a toe when she accidentally banged it on a chest of drawers. "Last year I wore sneakers all winter because of my ankle, and now I have to wear this slipper. I wonder what'll happen next."

She thinks it's only a matter of time until she has a major fracture, and although she's active, takes care of the house and her husband, and goes to work every day, she does worry about it. "I'm much more careful now. I've always loved to clean the house, and I climbed wherever I wanted to to wash the windows and whatnot, but now I have to change. Now, when I want to use the sweeper, John carries it upstairs, and when I'm finished, he carries it back down. But I still keep active. I'm on my feet a lot, running to the Xerox machine, going up and down stairs, and doing everything. I have an exercise bicycle that I use sometimes, although I *should* ride it every day."

She and John are thinking of moving even farther away from the city. It would be nice to have a smaller house for Roz to take care of and less polluted air for John to breathe. The suburb where they live now is congested but convenient, and they like where they live because they have friends there and are active in the local church and in community goings-on. So Roz and John find themselves in a dilemma: to stay where they are because they like it or move because it might be healthier for them.

Roz is a "typical" osteoporosis victim. She's white, was slight-of-build to begin with, and went through menopause when it wasn't commonly known that either estrogen and/or extra calcium could retard the disease. She has already lost a good deal of height and can break a toe just by bumping it into the furniture. But she's lucky because she's intelligent and is willing to do whatever she can to minimize the severity and the effects of the disease.

She's not assertive enough with her doctor, and in that respect she probably has much in common with other women her age. Roz is alert and aware enough to know what could possibly be in store for her, but she is also doing the best she can with a severe progressive disease.

* * *

Ruth Martin is not as lucky as Roz because not only is her osteoporosis far more advanced, but she has few of Roz's other advantages.

Ruth is so small—about 4 feet, 7 inches tall, and she probably weighs about 90 pounds—that a strong wind literally *could* knock her over. In fact, she does not venture outdoors when it's windy or when there's the least bit of ice or snow on the ground. She doesn't drive, but she lives across the street from a suburban mall (with a huge parking lot between, so it's probably more than a half-mile walk). It does her little good to live so close to the mall, though, because she hasn't the stamina to walk there and back.

Ruth is 77 years old, and her memory is fading fast. The last time she moved was in 1981, and she still can't remember her address. When the interview was arranged, she called twice to re-check the date, and even then she forgot about it. It's possible that she has the beginnings of Alzheimer's disease which, if true, will eventually cause even more serious problems.

Ruth can't remember when her bone troubles began, although from other things she said, it must be at least 20 years ago. She knows she's lost five inches of height, and she does remember the name of the disease. She also remembers to take her calcium tablets and the other medicines, "most of them for my head so I don't lose so much memory."

The loss of memory bothers her as much as the osteoporosis does, and the combination of the two makes life difficult and unpleasant. Sometimes she dreams that people are visiting her, and when she wakes up, she goes into the living room to discover that no one's there. Once she said she almost fell in the dark. Another time, "I called my daughter in the middle of the night and asked her where the boys [her grandchildren] were. I'd been dreaming that they were visiting me, and I got confused when I woke up."

The combination of a fuzzy memory and severe osteoporosis makes Ruth *almost* a shut-in. She lives in an apartment building for the elderly and takes advantage of many of the planned activities. For instance, she eats lunch every day in the community dining room. It serves as a "safety check" as well as her main meal; if she forgets to show up, someone knocks on her door. She also plays cards, games, and watches television with the other tenants in one of the community parlors.

Roz and John fetch her to and from church every Sunday, and other church friends drive her out shopping once in a while. "But I hate to impose on people like that. Sarah [her daughter] gets my groceries every Saturday, and sometimes she takes me out for a ride or to the store, but other than that, I don't go out much."

Ruth says she breaks a rib every now and then. When she hears one crack, all she has to do is lie down for a while; she doesn't even bother to go to the doctor about it. A broken rib usually requires more aggressive treatment than simple bed rest, so it's hard to know if she really is breaking ribs as often as she believes.

She's quite clear, however, about the pain along her spine, and judging by the amount of height she has lost and the severity of her kyphosis, it seems obvious that she has had several vertebral fractures and that she must be in a good deal of pain. She says the pain is intermittent, that sometimes it's worse than others. Sometimes two aspirin are enough, but more often she has to take something stronger. Bed rest seems to help, and if she lies down when the pain first begins, she can frequently prevent it from getting worse. Sometimes she uses a cane because her back hurts when she walks, and, "When I go to church, I have to roll my coat up and put it behind my back because it hurts to sit against those hard straight pews."

I asked Ruth what scares her the most about having osteoporosis.

"I'm afraid I'll fall. That really scares me. Actually I did fall once in the mall. Sarah was with me, and I was lucky that I didn't break anything, but ever since then I'm more afraid. I try to be awfully careful, and I use canes if I'm feeling off balance."

Ruth's life is pretty much circumscribed by the osteoporosis and to a lesser extent by her memory loss. She's mostly house-bound, except for short walks outside to get some fresh air in nice weather, and although she can't be described as a total cripple, she *is* old beyond her years. She gets around her apartment well and is independent enough to bathe, keep her home in order, and cook breakfast and a small supper for herself, but still, she's not a fully mobile person, and her independence has been severely curtailed.

She's lonely, especially at Christmas, and misses her husband who died 22 years ago at the end of December. At her daughter's insistence she moved east from her home in Kansas City when she began to grow frail, "because Sarah wanted me close so she could look after me." She moved four years ago to the government-subsidized apartment where she now lives because she could no longer afford the rent for her old apartment. Each time she moves, however, she leaves behind a support system and has to create a new one, which gets increasingly harder as she ages. This time, though, she found a built-in support system and has an opportunity to socialize every day at lunch and meet other elderly people with some of the same interests. It's not a horrible life, but neither is it as full and active as it could be, were it not for the osteoporosis.

Martha Hellman's condominium apartment is huge and sumptuously furnished. There are three bedrooms, two and a half bathrooms, a large balcony, and more closet space than any one person could possibly need. She has been living there alone for a decade, ever since she and her husband divorced. The apartment was part of the divorce settlement, and she's still collecting a healthy chunk of alimony every month—her "retirement pay," as she calls it.

Martha is 54 years old, although she looks much younger. About eight years ago, her doctor told her that she has "the bones of an 80-year-old woman." She has also lost an inch or two of height, but if you didn't know that, you'd never suspect that she has osteoporosis. She stands straight and erect and looked positively regal in her velvet hostess gown and perfectly coiffed hair, with makeup freshly and artfully applied. She had stayed home from work that day because of a cough, but she looked the picture of health in the evening.

Martha thinks she passed through menopause just within the past year but isn't sure because she had a hysterectomy when she was 37 for fibroid tumors that had caused unpleasantly heavy bleeding. It was the hot flashes and some of the other symptoms, which have just recently begun to subside, that made her think she was in menopause. She took estrogen replacement therapy for a short time, "But I hated it because I gained so much weight. So I stopped."

None of the research published about ERT indicates that weight gain is one of the side effects, but Martha insists that it happened to her. She knows that ERT is a good deterrent to osteoporosis, but she couldn't stand the idea of a few extra (and probably temporary) pounds.

"I'm one of those people who really hates to take medicine of any kind. I went to the library to read up on osteoporosis, and I read that despite everything and no matter how many medicines you take, there's no way to replace calcium in the bones. So I just decided not to do anything."

She does, however, take calcium pills but doesn't know how much of the mineral she gets every day because she doesn't know how much is in each tablet. Neither does she drink milk or eat cheese or yogurt because of the calories. Mostly she ignores the whole problem. "I just never think about my bones. I really sort of put it in the back of my head, and I've acted like it really isn't happening. I can break my bones pretty easily, though. It's almost embarrassing the way I break bones because practically every time someone hugs me, I can feel a rib crack." She also says she's broken her wrist once and her toes on several occasions.

Surely, she doesn't break her ribs that often. One of the reasons she's able to ignore the osteoporosis is because it doesn't hurt. But broken bones hurt, and if she has fractures as often as she says she does, surely, she must make the connection between the broken bones and the disease, which she seems to know a good deal about.

None of the doctors she sees regularly has much to say about her osteoporosis, "But I guess there's not much you can do about it—except exercise." Martha walks to and from her car, and she spends some time on her feet at work (she's the manager of a furniture showroom), but she has no regular exercise program.

She says that having osteoporosis doesn't affect her life much. Aside from taking some calcium, she says she doesn't think about it. But she's an intelligent woman who's read about the disease and has seen people with advanced cases. Thus, it's impossible to believe that behind that calm, self-assured façade, there isn't a very frightened woman.

Rose Keith is a tiny woman who describes herself as "all hips." It's not that her hips are especially wide, it's that her body configuration has changed so drastically that she has become unusually short-waisted, and her hips are indeed very close to her chest. She has a severe curvature, and she holds her head and neck at what appears to be an uncomfortable angle. She looks more crippled than she is, however, because she walks and moves with unexpected agility.

Rose is 70 now and has had osteoporosis for about 15 years. She first realized that something was drastically wrong when she picked up a small, relatively light coffee table and fractured a vertebra. The orthopedist who treated her back told her she had the disease and referred her to a gynecologist for hormones. "So I went to my own doctor, who put me on massive doses of some hormone [probably estrogen]. I took that for a while, but I just had more and more trouble."

Rose wore a brace for a while after she broke her back, longer than she now thinks she had to, but it didn't seem to help. "Then I began to have trouble with the upper part of my back, and that's because I was doing a very wrong thing. I would come home from work every day, lie down for a while, fix my dinner, and then go back in and lie down for the rest of the evening. Of course, now I know that the longer I stayed in bed, the worse things got. Eventually, I fractured several vertebrae up near my neck."

During the second broken vertebrae episode she was referred to an endocrinologist who got her started on an exercise program. She saw him periodically for about three years, and aside from taking occasional X-rays, he did little else. "He also put me on massive doses of another hormone, but I told him I couldn't continue to take them because I felt that my innards were going to drop right out of me."

All during this time her osteoporosis got worse, so she left the endocrinologist and embarked on what could be described only as a merry-go-round of nutritional programs which she continues to this day.

She has spent thousands of dollars and has gone to clinics,

doctors, and counselors from Boston to Wisconsin, each one espousing a slightly different philosophy of holistic health through nutrition. It's difficult to know, from the way Rose describes these programs, whether or not they are nutritionally sensible. Some sound more far out than others.

One doctor in Baltimore prescribed megavitamins and a vegetarian diet (although Rose cheated and ate some fish and poultry every now and again). After three years of this—and worsening osteoporosis—she left and went to an institute for preventive health. "There again I was on massive vitamin and mineral dosages. They did quite a bit with diet there. I stayed with that for about three years but was still losing height, and then I made a really bad decision. I went to a doctor and got six months of intravenous [directly into a vein] injections of calcium because this doctor said I'd never catch up with my calcium if I just took it in pill form. But I still kept losing height."

So she stopped that and went to yet another doctor, who injected some substance (an amino acid, she thought), again into her vein, that he said would "clean out" her blood vessels. What this has to do with osteoporosis is unclear, at least in Rose's mind, but she said she had read somewhere that this procedure would stimulate bone remineralization. "But it didn't do that for me."

Then she went to a clinic in Boston that claimed that raw food "would take care of all your ailments." She stayed there for two weeks but couldn't continue because she had trouble eating only raw fruits and vegetables. So she left the program and believes she failed, although she still grows her own "wheat grasses," sprouted sunflower seeds, and other kinds of freshly sprouted vegetation as instructed by the Boston clinic.

Even after all the money she has spent on these regimens, including buying special equipment that she believes she needs to sprout and grow things on her windowsills, nothing has helped her osteoporosis, and she has ended up feeling guilty about "failing" to improve. About the place in Boston, she said, "I know that people have been helped there. One man, a diabetic, told me about how he could stop taking insulin because his diabetes was completely cured. Other people were cured of heart disease and cancer. I know it works, but it was too much for me."

The sad thing is that Rose really does blame *herself* because she's not getting any better. Now, she is on a macrobiotic diet that a "nutrition counselor" recommended. Her feet swelled up and she had trouble walking, so she's had to modify the diet. But she sticks with it even though it doesn't do any good. She is now almost totally vegetarian and eats fish or poultry only once or twice a week unless she's invited to someone's house and there's nothing else to eat.

Research *has* shown that people with osteoporosis should avoid red meat, so she's on the right track there, but the rest of the diets that she's tried in the past—and will probably experiment with again in the future—will most likely do her no good, and all the excess vitamins she's taking can actually be harmful.

Rose has lost more than five inches of height. "You can't imagine how it is," she says, "to get on a bus and not be able to look out the window."

Her life has changed in other ways as well. Since she retired from a job where she sat at a desk all day (and drove to work), she has started to walk more; she tries to do a mile a day. Before she retired, she had a more active social life than she does now, but that meant that she spent little time at home cooking and lived mostly on prepared, processed food. Now she's careful of what she eats and how she cooks it. She buys only fresh food and sometimes even goes considerably out of her way to get organic produce.

Clothes are a major problem. "I can't buy clothes in a store, or if I do, they require major alterations. I try to make my own clothes, and I have scads of material here, but I never seem to have enough time."

Since last year, she hasn't been able to stand up straight, and she does exercises to strengthen her back muscles. But again, she feels as though she isn't trying hard enough. "I know there's a way to solve this problem [the osteoporosis], but I just haven't been able to find it, so I'll keep looking. Right now, I feel as though diet and exercise will be my salvation."

Rose really does believe there will eventually be "salvation" for her. She knows she can't have young bones again, but she thinks that if she could only find the right combination of diet and exercise, she could stop the bone loss.

Susie Everly lives at the end of what seems like the longest apartment building corridor in the city, and she uses it to her advantage. "Twelve round trips to the elevator equals two miles, and some days when it's too cold or nasty to go out, that's how I get my exercise."

Three years ago, she landed in the hospital after breaking her back, and that was when her osteoporosis was diagnosed. One of the doctors told her to walk two miles a day, and she has done so faithfully ever since.

She is 72 now (but has the face of a 50-year-old) and has broken vertebrae on three separate occasions. The first time, three years ago, she fractured two lumbar vertebrae but didn't realize it until the pain drove her into the hospital, where X-rays were taken, and the osteoporosis was first diagnosed. During that three-week hospitalization, she had a CAT scan and a complete neurological examination.

"I think they just wanted to use their machines and charge me for them," she says. "They didn't do anything for me."

She did have some physical therapy but now, as she looks back on the experience, she thinks she was kept in bed for far too long, and the prolonged inactivity was exactly the wrong thing for the doctors to have prescribed. "I was in traction, and only one nurse knew how to work the thing. Mostly, I had to put myself in and out of the contraption. And I was paying for all this!"

As she lay in the hospital, she started to worry about the future. "I asked the doctor if I was going to be a wheelchair patient for the rest of my life. Every time I'd ask that question, he'd leave the room. I think he didn't know the answer and was uncomfortable that I asked."

It was finally an endocrinologist who made the correct diagnosis, placed her on calcium supplements and Vitamin D and advised the two-mile-a-day walk. At first she walked only in the hallway where it's carpeted and safe because, "The pavement outdoors was so hard that every time I put my foot down, it jarred my back and hurt something awful. And I was scared crossing the street. I used to wait until the light had just turned green and then go as fast as I could, but the light would usually change before I got all the way across, and I was afraid I'd be run over."

Now that she's mostly out of pain, she goes out and about her business, but still sometimes she doesn't quite get across the street on the pedestrian signal. She's less afraid now of being in a wheelchair for the rest of her life, but she still thinks about it from time to time, especially if she's not feeling well one day. "I guess I'd have to go to a home somewhere because there's no way I could be independent. I've always had a dread of being in a wheelchair, and I'm grateful now that I can walk."

Susie has always been independent, and it would be hard for her to have to ask people to do physical things for her—even her roommate of 37 years. The two women have lived together since shortly after World War II, and although Susie didn't say so, it would be a wrench for them to be separated.

She drinks four glasses of skim milk every day, one of the few people interviewed who actually likes milk. She also eats cottage cheese and yogurt sometimes, and between her dietary intake and the supplemental pills, she gets about 3700 mg a day of calcium—more than twice what she needs. She also takes megadoses of Vitamin D—100,000 units a week. But she has no intention of cutting back on either the calcium or the Vitamin D, not only because the doctor prescribed it, but also because she believes in the "more is better" theory of medicine; that is, if a certain amount is good, then even more must be that much better.

Osteoporosis has changed Susie's life too. "I don't take trips any more unless I know that the destination will have a good bed. I have to have a very firm mattress and then I put a bedboard under it." She didn't know that practically all major hotels will provide a bedboard on request and seemed pleased to have this information.

She'll never travel overseas again because she can't sit for the long airplane ride (and sea travel is too expensive), and she doesn't ride for too long in a car. She was planning to fly to Florida, a two-hour plane ride, the day after the interview and worried about having enough legroom. She also didn't know that all airlines will reserve a seat in the front row of the cabin, so she can have all the legroom she needs.

Susie says she gets tired more easily than she used to, "Although part of that could be just old age." She carries nothing heavy and has bought a cart to get her groceries home from the supermarket. She wears flat-heeled shoes and has trouble with clothes. "All the height I've lost is in my body, but my legs are the same length, so I don't look nice in clothes. I wear slacks most of the time, and then it's not so noticeable that my body is out of proportion. But it's hard to look dressed up in low heels."

Susie does fewer things now, and she does them more slowly than she used to. She says ruefully, "I used to feel like a person. Now, I feel like an old woman."

She doesn't look like an old woman, though, and however much she has slowed down and curtailed some of her activities, her spirit remains young, and she has been able to preserve most of her independence. That's the important thing.

GLOSSARY

Adipose tissue—fat

Anatomy—study of body structures and their relationship to other structures

Androgen—a group of male hormones present in small amounts in females

Androstenedione—a form of androgen from which estrone is made by the process of aromatization

Aromatization—the process by which androstenedione is converted to estrone, most especially in adipose tissue

Biopsy—removal of a small sample of body tissue, preparation and staining of cells from that tissue, and examination of the cells under a microscope

Callus—a thick horny layer of skin or other tissue; the osseous material, composed of cartilage and other tissue, formed between bone fragments of a healing fracture

Cardiovascular—pertaining to the heart and blood vessels

Cartilage—a type of dense connective tissue, some of which always exists in a cartilaginous state and some of which converts to bone

Central nervous system—combination of the brain and spinal cord

Cervical spine—the top 7 of the 33 spinal vertebrae

Cholesterol—a form of alcohol widely found in animal tissues; the principal component of gallstones; a precursor to various sex hormones

Coccygeal spine—the 4 vertebrae at the end of the spine

Comminution—displacement of bone fragments; nonalignment of fragments

Cortical bone *(substantia corticalis)*—a dense compacted mass of bone tissue that forms the external covering layer of bones

Edema—tissue swelling

Embolism—a blood clot that travels to another part of the body

Endometrium—the lining of the uterus to which the fertilized ovum attaches and which sloughs off each month the ovum is not fertilized

Endosteal envelope—the layer of bone closest to the marrow cavity

Estradiol—one type of estrogen, produced in the ovary

Estrogen—the group of female hormones responsible for the appearance and maintenance of secondary sex characteristics, ovulation, and other uniquely female functions

Estrone—a form of estrogen converted from androgen

Extension—pulling both ends of a part in opposite directions

Flexion—the act of bending

Hematoma—a blood clot

Hypertension—high blood pressure

Hysterectomy—surgical removal of the uterus

Intracortical envelope—the middle layer of bone

Kyphosis—excessive curvature of the upper spine, commonly called humpback

Lumbar spine—the 5 vertebrae in the lower back

Marrow—the substance contained within the hollow center of long bones in which white and red blood cells, platelets, and other blood components are formed

Menopause—cessation of menstruation; a full year after the last menstrual period; occurs between age 45 and 55

Metabolism—the sum of all physical and chemical changes within an organism; all energy and material transformations that occur within cells

Necrosis—death and decay of tissue

Neurologist—a physician who specializes in the nervous system

Nutrient—a food or food substance that supplies the body with the elements required for metabolism

Oophorectomy—surgical removal of an ovary

Orthopedist (orthopod)—a physician who specializes in the treatment of bone and joint diseases and injuries

Osteoblast—a cell that creates bone

Osteoclast—a cell that destroys bone

Osteomalacia—delayed or diminished mineralization of new bone

Osteopenia—decreased volume of mineralized bone

Ovary—one of a pair of structures, about the size and shape of an almond, where estrogen is produced, where ova are stored, and from which an ovum is released each month

Ovum—a unicellular female egg

Parathyroid—the pea-sized endocrine gland located next to, or embedded in, the thyroid; secretes parathyroid hormone that regulates metabolism of calcium and phosphorus

Periosteal envelope—the outer layer of bone

Physiology—study of function; how anatomical structures work

Progestogen (commonly called progesterone)—another group of female hormones, this one responsible primarily for the buildup of the endometrium and its preparation for receipt of the fertilized ovum

Prophylaxis—prevention

Reduction—the process of fitting fractured bone fragments together and then immobilizing them until the fracture heals

Remodeling—the process of buildup and breakdown of bone tissue that continues, at varying rates, throughout life

Risk factor—a factor that will increase the chance of something happening; i.e., smoking is a risk factor for lung cancer

Sacral spine—the 5 vertebrae at the top of the buttocks

Thoracic spine—the middle 12 of the 33 spinal vertebrae

Trabecular bone *(spongiosa)*—the latticelike inner layer of spongy bone that derives its strength from its intricate architecture

Traction—applying weight to one end of a bone, while holding the other end steady, to extend it and hold it in place

APPENDIX:
PAIN CLINICS

Baptist Hospital
Miami, Florida 33176

City of Hope Medical Center
Los Angeles, California 90052

Johns Hopkins University Hospital
Baltimore, Maryland 21205

Mensana Clinic
Stevenson, Maryland 21153

Mount Sinai Hospital
Miami, Florida 33140

New York University Medical Center
New York, New York 10016

Rush Presbyterian–St. Luke's Medical Center
Chicago, Illinois 60612

Scripps Clinics
Claremont, California 91711

University of Illinois Hospital
Chicago, Illinois 60612

University of Washington Medical Center
Seattle, Washington 98105

Our Lady of Lourdes Hospital
Binghamton, New York 13905

Cox Pain Center
San Luis Obispo, California 93401

Massachusetts General Hospital
Boston, Massachusetts 02114

Del Oro Hospital
Houston, Texas 77002

University of Virginia Medical Center
Charlottesville, Virginia 22901

Emory University Hospital
Atlanta, Georgia 30322

University of Pittsburgh Medical Center
Pittsburgh, Pennsylvania 15261

University of California Medical Center
Los Angeles, California 90024

For further information:

American Medical Association
Washington, D.C. 20005

NOTES

CHAPTER 1 Osteoporosis: What It Is

1. Z. F. G. Jaworski, "Physiology and Pathology of Bone Remodeling," in ed. J. Menczel, et al., *Osteoporosis: The Proceeding of an International Symposium Held at the Jerusalem Osteoporosis Center in June, 1981* (Chichester, England: John Wiley, 1982) 485.

2. Joseph Melton and Laurence Riggs, "Evidence for Two Distinct Syndromes of Involutional Osteoporosis," *American Journal of Medicine* 75(6) (Dec. 1983), 899–901.

3. Ibid.

4. Ibid.

CHAPTER 2 Diagnosis and Treatment

1. C. Conrad Johnston and Solomon Epstein, "Clinical Features of Osteoporosis," in ed. Harold M. Frost, "Symposium of the Osteoporoses," *The Orthopedics Clinics of North America* 12(3) (Philadelphia: W. B. Saunders, July, 1981) 564.

2. Ibid.

3. Harold M. Frost, ed., "Symposium on the Osteoporoses," *The Orthopedic Clinics of North America* 12(3) (Philadelphia: W. B. Saunders, July 1981) 604.

4. Ibid., 608–09.

5. Robert R. Recker, "Continuous Treatment of Osteoporosis: Current Status," in *Frost,* 616.

6. Ibid.

7. Ibid.

8. Ibid.

9. *Frost,* "Symposium on the Osteoporoses," 674–75.

CHAPTER 3 Estrogen Replacement Therapy

1. N. Kreiger, et al., "An Epidemiologic Study of Hip Fracture in Postmenopause Women," *American Journal of Epidemiology* 116 (July, 1982).

2. B. S. Hulka, L. E. Chambless, et al., "Breast Cancer and Estrogen Replacement Therapy," *American Journal of Obstetrics and Gynecology* 143 (July 15, 1982).

3. P. D. Saville, "Post-menopausal Osteoporosis and Estrogen: Who Should Be Treated and Why," *Postgraduate Medicine* 75 (Feb. 1, 1985).

4. A. Horsman, M. Jones, et al., "The Effect of Estrogen Dose on Postmenopausal Bone Loss," *The New England Journal of Medicine* 309 (Dec. 8, 1983) 152.

5. Clare D. Erdman, "The Climacteric," in ed. Herbert J. Bushman, *The Menopause* (New York: Springer-Verlag, 1983) 152.

6. Ibid.

7. Ibid.

CHAPTER 4   Fractures

1. R. Bruce Heppenstall, *Fracture Treatment and Healing* (Philadelphia: W. B. Saunders, 1980) 340.

2. Ibid.

3. Ibid.

4. Ibid.

5. Ibid.

REFERENCES

Biegel, Leonard, ed. *Physical Fitness and the Older Person: A Guide to Exercise for Health Care Professionals.* Rockville, Md.: Aspen Systems Corp., 1984.

Christiansen, C., et al. "Does Postmenopausal Bone Loss Respond to Estrogen Replacement Therapy Independent of Bone Loss Rate?" *Calcification Tissue International.* September, 1983. 35:720–22.

DeLuca, H. F., et al., eds. *Osteoporosis: Recent Advances in Pathogenesis and Treatment.* Baltimore: University Park Press, 1981.

Erdman, Clare D. "The Climacteric," in Buchsbaum, Herbert J., ed. *The Menopause.* New York: Springer-Verlag, 1983.

Fritz, Marc and Leon Speroff. "Role of Progestational Agents in Hormone Replacement Therapy," in *Buchsbaum.*

Frost, Harold M., ed. "Symposium on the Osteoporoses," *The Orthopedic Clinics of North America.* Vol. 12: no. 3. Philadelphia: W. B. Saunders. July 1983.

Heppenstall, R. Bruce. *Fracture Treatment and Healing.* Philadelphia: W. B. Saunders, 1980.

Horsman, A., M. Jones, et al. "The Effect of Estrogen Dose on Postmenopausal Bone Loss," *The New England Journal of Medicine.* December 8, 1983. 390:1405–07.

Hulka, B. S., L. E. Chambless, et al. "Breast Cancer and Estrogen Replacement Therapy," *American Journal of Obstetrics and Gynecology.* July 15, 1982. 143:638–44.

Jaworski, Z. F. G. "Physiology and Pathology of Bone Remodeling," in *Menczel.*

Johnston, C. Conrad, and Solomon Epstein. "Clinical Features of Osteoporosis," in *Frost.*

Kreiger, N., et al. "An Epidemiologic Study of Hip Fracture in Postmenopausal Women," *American Journal of Epidemiology.* July, 1982. 116:141–48.

Melton, Joseph, and Laurence Riggs. "Evidence for Two Distinct Syndromes of Involutional Osteoporosis," *American Journal of Medicine.* December, 1983. 75(6):899–901.

Menczel, J., et al., eds. *Osteoporosis: The Proceedings of an International Symposium Held at the Jerusalem Osteoporosis Center in June 1981*. Chichester, England: John Wiley, 1982.

Nordin, B. E. C. "Osteoporosis," in *Wright*.

Pollock, Michael L., Jack H. Wilmore and Samuel M. Fox III. *Exercise in Health and Disease*. Philadelphia: W. B. Saunders, 1984.

Recker, Robert R. "Continuous Treatment of Osteoporosis: Current Status," in *Frost*.

Saville, P. D. "Post-menopausal Osteoporosis and Estrogens: Who Should Be Treated and Why," *Postgraduate Medicine*. February 1, 1984. 75:135–38, 142–43.

Sherman, B., and R. Wallace, et al. "Estrogen Use and Breast Cancer: Interaction with Body Mass," *Cancer*. April 15, 1983. 51:1527–31.

Skinner, Alison T., and Ann M. Thomson. *Duffield's Exercise in Water*. 3rd ed. East Sussex, England: Baillière Tindall, 1983.

Turek, Samuel L., *Orthopaedics*. 4th ed. Philadelphia: J. B. Lippincott, 1984.

Wright, V., ed. *Bone and Joint Disease in the Elderly*. Edinburgh: Churchill Livingstone, 1983.

INDEX